T0291053

First Principles

First Principles

Applied Ethics for Psychoanalytic Practice

Alessandra Lemma

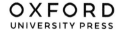

OXFORD
UNIVERSITY PRESS

OXFORD
UNIVERSITY PRESS

Great Clarendon Street, Oxford, OX2 6DP,
United Kingdom

Oxford University Press is a department of the University of Oxford.
It furthers the University's objective of excellence in research, scholarship,
and education by publishing worldwide. Oxford is a registered trade mark of
Oxford University Press in the UK and in certain other countries

© Oxford University Press 2023

The moral rights of the author have been asserted

First Edition published in 2023

All rights reserved. No part of this publication may be reproduced, stored in
a retrieval system, or transmitted, in any form or by any means, without the
prior permission in writing of Oxford University Press, or as expressly permitted
by law, by licence or under terms agreed with the appropriate reprographics
rights organization. Enquiries concerning reproduction outside the scope of the
above should be sent to the Rights Department, Oxford University Press, at the
address above

You must not circulate this work in any other form
and you must impose this same condition on any acquirer

Published in the United States of America by Oxford University Press
198 Madison Avenue, New York, NY 10016, United States of America

British Library Cataloguing in Publication Data
Data available

Library of Congress Control Number: 2022950787

ISBN 978–0–19–285896–2

DOI: 10.1093/med-psych/9780192858962.001.0001

Printed and bound by
CPI Group (UK) Ltd, Croydon, CR0 4YY

Oxford University Press makes no representation, express or implied, that the
drug dosages in this book are correct. Readers must therefore always check
the product information and clinical procedures with the most up-to-date
published product information and data sheets provided by the manufacturers
and the most recent codes of conduct and safety regulations. The authors and
the publishers do not accept responsibility or legal liability for any errors in the
text or for the misuse or misapplication of material in this work. Except where
otherwise stated, drug dosages and recommendations are for the non-pregnant
adult who is not breast-feeding

Links to third party websites are provided by Oxford in good faith and
for information only. Oxford disclaims any responsibility for the materials
contained in any third party website referenced in this work.

To my patients, with gratitude

Acknowledgements

My patients have been some of my best teachers and I am grateful for the learning.

I am deeply indebted to Andy Law for his expert knowledge of ancient Greek and Latin, for sharing my love of etymology and for accommodating with generosity and love my preoccupation with this book. I want to thank Heather Wood and Linda Young for their encouragement and very helpful comments on earlier drafts. Their wisdom, curiosity, and friendship have been invaluable.

I could not have engaged with the themes I develop in the pages to come were it not for the excellent teaching in applied ethics that I was privileged to receive at the *Uheiro Centre for Ethics* at Oxford University. I am indebted to all the philosophers and ethicists whose thinking has encouraged me to think more and, I hope, to also 'think better', at least some of the time.

Finally, I want to thank Routledge for permission to reprint adapted clinical sections from A. Lemma (2022) 'Transgender Identities' and A. Lemma (2013) 'Transference on the Couch'. In: R. Olser (ed.) *Transference and Countertransference Today*.

Contents

"Do you feel no compunction, Socrates, at having fol-lowed a line of action which puts you in danger of the death penalty?"

I might fairly reply to him, "You are mistaken, my friend, if you think that a man who is worth anything ought to spend his time weighing up the prospects of life and death. He has only one thing to consider in performing any action—that is, whether he is acting rightly or wrongly, like a good man or a bad one."

—Socrates, Apology

Introduction: Living the Questions

One of my favourite pieces from Rilke's collection of *Letters to a Young Poet* (1929) is the 1903 letter to Franz Xaver Kappus, himself an aspiring poet, who turned to Rilke for advice. In this impassioned response, Rilke writes:

> I should like to ask you . . . to be patient toward all that is unsolved in your heart and to try to love the *questions themselves* like locked rooms, like books written in a foreign tongue. Do not now strive to uncover answers, they cannot be given you because you have not been able to live them . . . and what matters is to live everything. Perhaps you will then gradually, without noticing it, live your way into the answer. (1929: 17; italics in the original)

I draw your attention to Rilke's quote because I want to invite you, the reader, to *love* and *live the questions* as you read this book. Questions are challenging because they can take us to new places in our minds, but this requires letting go of ideas or beliefs to which we have become married. Our willingness to suspend knowing, to relinquish the comforts of certainty, to open ourselves to that which we have not yet thought, is vital to our work. The ability to think independently, with the courage to openly question established wisdom and one's own conceptual footholds and prejudices, is also the backbone of ethical practice. Wilfred Bion was not discussing ethics, but he grasped the vital necessity of questions:

> Experience brings it home to you that you can give what we call 'answers' but they are really space stoppers. It is a way of putting an end to curiosity—especially if you succeed in believing the answer is *the* answer. (Bion, 1978: 22, italics in original)

Questions are the life blood of ethical practice. As human beings, we are drawn to certainties. We have been adept at seeking out echo chambers feeding back to us self-confirmatory information and re-assurance well before technology used algorithms to support this human need and vulnerability. This should not surprise us: our narcissism is the shared human Achilles' heel. We seek to be mirrored. Difference is often threatening. Alterity presents as a question that demands our self-focus to give way to what is 'not-me'. The best questions expose us to what is unfamiliar, to 'not-me', inviting us to imagine the person who is different to us. To welcome questions, I am therefore suggesting, is to welcome the disruption introduced by otherness. However, 'imagining' otherness (Scarry, 1998) in-variably mobilizes a universally shared relational ambivalence. We spend our lives carefully choreographing (mostly unconsciously) a tolerable position in relation to the 'other' on the related axes of proximity-distance and sameness-difference. Ethical choice presents itself when we are faced with someone or something that threatens to destabilize our relational choreography and the world as we know it, something that disturbs the taken-for-granted coordinates of our daily lives and sense of who we are. Otherness is disruptive in this fundamental sense. It is precisely when we face this kind of 'disrup-tion' that we are also confronted with our ethics.

Stepping out of the cave

Francis Bacon (1889) laid out the foundations of modern sciences in *Novum Organum*. The ideas he presented in this work are pre-scient to the focus of this book because Bacon's doctrine of 'idols' touched on the dangers that ensue when our narcissism impels us to deny otherness and difference. He described four idols[1] through which he exposed his understanding of the various obstacles that get in the way of truth-false idols that prevent us from making accurate

---

[1] The four idols are: Idols of the Tribe, Idols of the Cave, Idols of the Marketplace, and Idols of the Theatre. I am only focusing on 'Idols of the Cave'.

observations and achieving understanding. Bacon's '*idols of the cave*'[2] (1889: 21) are especially relevant to ethical practice, and I selectively focus on these, because they refer to the problems that result from our passions and enthusiasms, our devotions, and ideologies.

For Bacon, our 'cave' refracts the light of truth, owing either to our idiosyncrasies, education, allegiances, or the authority of those whom we esteem and admire. These, I suggest, function as blind spots, and potentially work against ethical practice. Psychoanalytically speaking, our internal objects inhabit the cave that is our unconscious and this introduces another source of bias. Ethical practice requires us to step out of this cave too, in so far as that is possible, and be prepared to attend to our unconscious and its trappings. It thus requires that we strive to relinquish the comforts of conscious and unconscious idols—this is an aspiration and not a state that we can reach and sustain in any absolute way because, by definition, the unconscious cannot be mastered. At best we can be curious about our 'idols of the cave' and learn more about our recurrent patterns and traps so that more of the time we can attend to their impact on our mind and on our relationships, not least the relationship we develop with each of our patients. The resistances we meet in the process of stepping out of the cave are not only intrapsychic ones. Institutional resistances also operate and complicate this process. A training institution and its system(s), which cannot be neatly separated out from the wider cultural systems in which it is embedded, can also function as a cave as much as our own blind spots can obfuscate our understanding of who we are and of the other. Ethical practice therefore involves being prepared to not only challenge ourselves but also the wider systems that frame our clinical practice.

I first turned to ethics when I was grappling with understanding two clinical issues: the increase in referrals of young people identifying as transgender and the impact on psychic functioning of our interface with digital technologies. Psychoanalysis provided an essential backbone to my clinical work. But making sense of my

---

[2] He also refers to these as idols of the 'den' or 'cavern'.

responsibility as a therapist facing these sociocultural changes at the intersection of the individual psyche, required something more. It necessitated stepping out of the cave of my first and much-loved conceptual psychoanalytic home. The 'something more', for me, proved to be applied ethics.[3] My 'ethical turn', as it were, was therefore initially prompted by some of the challenges that I faced in the consulting room and not by a concern with how the psychoanalytic profession addressed the ethics of clinical practice in a more general sense. However, as I studied ethics, it became clear to me that during psychoanalytic training we are underprepared for addressing the ethics of psychoanalytic practice. Beyond a handful of seminars, thinking about ethics appears to be considered an implicit function of supervision with only very limited explicit conceptualization of the place of ethics in our work. This book concerns itself with the articulation of one conceptual framework that can sustain us to do our best for our patients.

I must own up: I find frameworks and models appealing because they help me to organize my thinking. I recognize that they are imperfect creations, always falling short, because we can never reduce the mind, or the vicissitudes of the encounter between two subjectivities, to a schema or diagram. Models risk becoming yet another cave that blinds us. Even so, I think they have some modest value, not least for those who are tasked with a training function and for those who are in training. That said, the rational approach of applied ethics to addressing often emotive clinical dilemmas may jar at first. It does not easily reconcile itself with what we know instinctively about the complex and sometimes messy reality of the analytic relationship (well, of any relationship) and the risks to which it exposes both participants. The nuances and the passion can never be adequately captured in the rational philosophical terms that attempt to bring some order to bear on the process. And, yet, I will argue, there is merit in learning from the field of applied ethics and its disciplined approach to thinking.

---

[3] See Glossary for definition.

The ideas that I share in this book are rooted in 35 years of clinical and teaching experience as a social worker first, then as a clinical psychologist, later still as a psychoanalyst, and most recently in applied ethics. As such, this book is idiosyncratic. I have approached its content in the spirit of starting a conversation in our discipline with an explicit training agenda: how can we train therapists in such a way that we reduce the risk of ethical breaches and are better equipped to manage when breaches or errors do occur? There is, of course, the equally important question of how we can improve the way that patients can be supported when they must make a complaint about a therapist. This is not the focus of this book, but it is a vital question. Indeed, the impetus for this book has also been propelled by the painful experiences reported to me by some of my patients and that I have heard about through supervision of other colleagues' work. At their most vulnerable, these individuals entrusted their minds to psychotherapists and were met instead with sexual and psychic intrusion. Sadly, such instances are not as rare as we might like to believe. The fact that our ethics committees are not inundated with such complaints is not evidence of the absence or infrequency of such transgressions. Rather, it reflects how difficult, if not impossible, it can be for some patients to take the step to complain. As we know from cases of sexual assault or coercive mental control outside of our own discipline, many women (and it is mostly women) never come forward. The reluctance to do so can be understood in many ways but it is especially complicated when the perpetrator is known to the person and often is a figure of attachment on whom the victim continues to depend or has depended upon. The decision to not pursue a complaint against a therapist may reflect a fear of not being believed and of being exposed through a (costly) legal process that will play on their unreliability as witnesses because of the mental health problems that led them to seek therapy in the first place. It may also speak to the poignant complexities of the transference to a therapist who is both loved, feared and/or hated in equal measure, and this prevents the patient from taking forward a complaint.

Psychoanalysis and ethics

When I began to study ethics, I experienced the surge of excitement that I always encounter when I discover new ideas—ones that invite different questions and open 'locked rooms', as Rilke surmised. Interdisciplinary thinking is energizing. Ethics and psychoanalysis need each other. Without the conceptual tools to think about ethics, the psychoanalytic therapist runs the risk of operating only intuitively, with the attendant limitations of such an approach. Intuition alone or being well-intentioned do not necessarily result in making sound decisions when we face clinical dilemmas or when we consider the ethics of our own daily practice, which is why psychoanalysis needs ethics. In turn, ethics needs psychoanalysis because a conceptualization of basic ethical principles (e.g. autonomy) is diminished if we fail to consider an agent who has an unconscious mind.[4]

This book's main objective is to make the case for the centrality of applied ethics to psychoanalytic practice specifically. I do not address the formal questions that concern meta-ethics (i.e. the assumptions that underpin normative judgements such as 'what is goodness?') or the substantive questions that preoccupy normative ethics (i.e. how we ought to act) and that coalesce around specific moral theories such as utilitarianism or deontology.[5] I am therefore not concerned with the articulation of a conception of what constitutes a 'good' life or a 'good' character per se. Rather, I focus on the importance of developing and exercising an identifiable method—an ethical self-discipline—to support critical reflection on our daily work with patients and to help us when we face ethical dilemmas. As such, this book is not intended to be a comprehensive or critical overview of applied ethics philosophically or clinically.

I am primarily concerned with the ethics of the individual psychoanalytic therapist and the ethics of psychoanalysis as a method. The ethical specificity of psychoanalysis is determined by its method

---

[4] One of the areas that I do not address in this book is how consideration of any range of bioethical dilemmas can itself benefit from psychoanalytic concepts (to get a sense of this kind of application, see Appel, 2011).
[5] See Glossary for a definition.

(Donnet, 2011; Glass, 2021; Scarfone, 2017), by which I mean that the method relies on the active use of the analytic relationship. I will only briefly touch on the question of whether psychoanalysis should be helping people to act morally or be more virtuous[6] or with how psychotherapeutic progress in therapy might itself be construed as ethical in nature.[7] These are very important questions but to do them justice, they deserve another book. Instead, my focus is more modest and circumscribed: to set out a framework to support the reflective process that is the essential underpinning of applied ethics to psychoanalytic work. To this end I draw on the four prima facie principles of bioethics (Beauchamp and Childress, 2013), and I reinterpret them within a psychoanalytic frame, applying them to the specificity of the analytic encounter.

The position I set out in this book is based on several presumptions about how I understand the analytic process and what distinguishes it from other types of therapy. I do not articulate a defence of these presumptions—that constitutes a different piece of work that is beyond the remit of my focus here. As therapists, we must each come to our own answers about the purpose of psychoanalytic work, using our preferred moral and psychoanalytic theories, or possibly argue that morality has nothing to do with psychoanalysis. I will not enter these debates in any detail. However, I suggest that we cannot offer a form of help for the mind without at the same time considering a set of common moral commitments such as those provided by the core ethical principles I outline.

Our interventions always have an ethical dimension; that is, they fundamentally concern doing what is best for the patient. *Applied ethics* refers to the implementation of a systematic, deliberative approach to making clinical judgements that retains the focus on what is best for the patient rather than being hijacked, for example, by the therapist's allegiance to her favoured theory of psychic health. It is about helping us to think more truthfully (McCoy Brooks, 2013) so that we can arrive at a considered position about what to do in a

---

[6] To get a flavour for the debate, see Harcourt (2018) and Groacke (2018).
[7] See Drozek (2019) and Wallwork (1991) for helpful discussions of these themes.

certain set of circumstances. This process engages our ethical conscience. Erik Erickson provides the most articulate distinction that I have come across between a moral and ethical conscience:

> Developmentally speaking we must, in fact, differentiate between an earlier, a *moral* conscience and a later, an *ethical* one. What Freud graphically calls our superego, that part of our conscience which forever lords it over us and at times seems to crush us with guilt, serves as the internalization of early prohibitions driven into us by frowning faces and verbal threats . . . . In later life, this remains our most moralistic side—that side of us which takes pleasure in condemning those who are doing what we could not dare to do and, so we claim, are endangering the moral fibre of mankind. The more *adult* pole of our ethical nature is an affirmative sense of what man owes to man, in terms of the developmental realization of the best in each human being. (Erikson, 1976: 413, italics in original)

I have been using the word 'ethics' mindful that it can sound all too abstract. Yet, when Aristotle differentiated ἦθος ethos (character) from διάνοιά dianoia (intellect), he reminds us that when we are talking about ethics, we are not then talking about something lofty or abstract. We are, first and foremost, talking about 'us', and the 'us' that concerns me in this book are the people who choose to practice a form of help that we call psychoanalysis. Ethics cannot be something apart from us, a set of rules we abide by or fall short of. It is about *how* we approach our work, and this reveals who we are as people. At its core, the ethical impulse rests on a commitment to see the world through another's eyes.[8] We can only honour this commitment if we can tolerate looking at who we are, not least when we get things wrong. This is both an individual responsibility but, as I shall argue, it is also the responsibility of the institutions that train us and support our ongoing professional development once we qualify. We need to create a space within trainings, psychoanalytic societies, and

---

[8] This is not the same as agreeing with the other person—it is about receptivity to, and respect for, different viewpoints and the reality of difference.

ultimately in our own mind for thinking critically about our work as individuals and as a discipline.

Inevitably, writing about ethics can give the impression that the author knows better and is somehow 'holier than thou' addressing colleagues who have much to learn in this respect. I hope that I have managed to describe and discuss the challenges we are all faced with in our work, and the risks inherent to it, without straying into becoming an analytic superego or succumbing to virtue signalling.

About this book

This is a book of two halves. The first part, Chapters 1–4, is conceptual and sets the scene for the more applied chapters. Knowledge of key psychoanalytic ideas is assumed, but there is no assumption of prior knowledge of applied ethics. Chapter 2 provides a brief overview of key ethical principles aimed at clinicians with little or no knowledge of ethics and there is a Glossary at the end of the book of some key terms. A word of caution: if you are not well versed in ethics, skipping the first four chapters will likely result in frustration and disappointment as you reach for the second half of the book. The latter assumes that you are by then acquainted with the arguments of the book, with the core ethical principles derived from bioethics and how I have interpreted these for psychoanalytic consumption. The second part, Chapters 5–8, is more applied to clinical work and outlines the training implications of the arguments I set out. The book is aimed at all psychoanalytic colleagues irrespective of the frequency or length of their analytic work, and hence I focus on generalities rather than the specifics of one type of analytic modality.

In Chapter 1, I define the responsible therapist as the one who makes a unique 'psychoanalytic promise' to the patient: I will allow you to 'use' me, within the boundaries of the analytic setting, to serve your best interests in developing a mind of your own. This promise can only be kept if we maintain a horizontal relationship with the patient, that is a structurally similar relationship of equals, and ensure that it does not become a malignant vertical relationship where we abuse the asymmetrical power that is inherent in our role within the analytic relationship. This requires us to be alert to the fact that the therapist (i.e. not only the patient) inevitably impacts the analytic process through her needs, desires, anxieties, and defences. We need to closely monitor how we influence the process precisely because analytic work is mediated by us. I suggest therefore that the development of the analytic attitude—the cornerstone of analytic work—needs to be articulated in relation to what I term the *ethical chóros*.[1] This denotes a *principled internal space* that regulates our practice through supporting self-questioning in relation to our work and the obligations we have towards our patients, the most fundamental of which is that we must create and safeguard in our mind a dwelling space for the patient and his singularity. The ethical chóros is the part of our internal setting that monitors the tensions arising from the confrontation with our responsibility for the other and the defences this can mobilize, as well the ethical breaches or errors we can succumb to. If we believe in an unconscious mind, we know that it is precisely because of its existence that the analytic endeavour cannot but be subject at times to errors or ethical breaches of different magnitudes—a theme that will be developed in the book. Of course, we both know this and may choose not to know it.

Chapter 2 introduces the dominant model used in bioethics: the Four Principles approach as described by Beauchamp and Childress (2013). I suggest that this provides a helpful base model to support our practice and do our best by the patient. This chapter is a highly condensed introduction to the four principles of bioethics.[2] I assume these principles rather than argue for them, namely respect for autonomy (the obligation to respect the decision-making capacities of autonomous persons); non-maleficence (the obligation to avoid causing harm); beneficence (the obligation to provide benefits and to balance benefits against risks); and justice (the obligation of fairness). I propose that we use these not only as a method for reflecting on specific ethical dilemmas but also as important checkpoints for reflecting on our daily practice.

Chapter 3 builds on the Four Principles model and reinterprets it for use by psychoanalytic clinicians. I add a fifth principle—veracity—that is integral to psychoanalytic work. I begin with a discussion of the *telos* of psychoanalytic therapy (i.e. its purpose).

[1] From the Greek, χῶρος meaning a clearly defined space/environment/dwelling space. This is quite different from a 'chorus' (χορός), a band of singers and dancers, even though it is phonetically similar.
[2] See Glossary for definition.

I suggest that addressing the question 'what is psychoanalysis for?' is fundamental, and even though there is no 'right' answer, articulating our idiosyncratic answer to this question is an essential requirement to working ethically. If we cannot articulate what we are offering or that we think that we are offering (I say this because there can be a striking difference between what we think and say we do and what we actually do), or we claim that we are not concerned with such matters, this is an ethical red flag. We cannot safely offer a professional encounter and not be prepared to engage with what it is that we think we do *for* the patient. Neither is it ethical to *only* respond to the question posed by a patient about 'How will this help me?' with an invitation to elaborate on his anxieties and fantasies about starting therapy. We offer a form of psychological help, and we are accountable for what we believe we can offer and how it might or might not benefit the patient.

In approaching the challenge of finding some common ground about the purpose of psychoanalytic work given the theoretical diversity in psychoanalysis, I draw on two sets of experiences. First, the work I carried out with colleagues in 2008 distilling the core competences for the practice of psychoanalytic therapy (Lemma et al., 2008). Second, I draw on the work as Independent Chair of the SCoPEd project (Scope of Practice and Education)—a three-year project that was completed at the end of 2021.[3] This latter focused on the development of an evidence-based framework to inform the training requirements, competences and ethical practice standards for counsellors and psychotherapists in the UK. Pulling together three psychotherapy registering bodies representing around 60,000 counsellors and psychotherapists in the UK from different schools of thought (e.g. humanistic, psychoanalytic, and so on), with different agendas and value systems, as a working group we had to be transparent about our process and prioritize our responsibilities to the public. Many outstanding colleagues contributed to this mammoth task, and credit goes to them for the final output.

---

[3] Available at: https://www.bacp.co.uk/about-us/advancing-the-profession/scoped/scoped-framework. Accessed 20 July 2022.

I share these experiences because they provide a background context for understanding the stance from which I approach this book: I write for psychoanalytic colleagues and as a practicing clinician but one informed by experiences that many psychoanalysts and psychoanalytic therapists are not typically involved in and may even be wary of. The language of 'competences', of 'operationalizing' what we do, is not to everyone's taste and may even be deemed by some to be inappropriate to the nature of the analytic endeavour. Capturing the complex, nuanced nature of the analytic encounter is indeed a challenge. Although I am sympathetic to the view that a list of competences, for example, falls short of this challenge, nevertheless it makes some inroads that allow us to represent our work to others—not least the public who use psychotherapy services and those who hold the money for publicly funded mental health provision—in a more transparent manner. Transparency is fundamental to ethical practice. It is not possible to meaningfully consent to a therapeutic process that cannot be described and understood by the layperson. Lest the mere mention of the word 'competences' leads you to decide this book is not for you, let me reassure you that I am not focusing here on competences. I am merely owning the conceptual baggage that informs my view of our profession and how I think it can improve further.

In Chapter 4, I consider the ethical complexity of listening. Drawing on the work of the philosopher Emmanuel Levinas, I suggest that the essence of ethical listening involves preparedness for the 'Other', but this otherness always demands something that conflicts with the therapist's desire[4] and narcissism. The Other primarily demands space in our mind. This is what the therapist promises to offer but even in the best of circumstances, at some stage, we will fall short of this promise because narcissism is not a developmental phase—it is a permanent feature of being human. The potential for iatrogenic effects is therefore significant, no matter how 'well analysed' we are or think we are.

---

[4] Desire is used here to refer both to the therapist's sexual desire and to their non-sexual desires.

Acting ethically relies on our willingness to question ourselves and to recognize that, even if only in minor ways, we all act unethically at least some of the time. The question is not if, but when and how. This reality gets overshadowed by the focus on major transgressions. We must address these instances of gross misconduct. However, such a narrow focus allows us as a discipline to fade into the shadow of the outliers and ignore our own more quotidian transgressions (Slochower, 2003). It is always reassuring to locate the problem elsewhere, or as Muriel Dimen (2011) put it, to get rid of the 'rotten apple' rather than recognizing that without due care, we can all be 'rotten' in different ways and to different degrees, some of the time. Chapter 5 therefore focuses on how we can think about different forms of 'getting it wrong' and I consider some specific psychoanalytic occupational hazards. In Chapter 6, I then explore what constitutes an ethical response 'when things go wrong'. I discuss the Duty of Candour and the function of the apology.

By way of an illustration of applied ethics, in Chapter 7 I share some clinical examples. I focus in some detail on my experience of how an applied ethics approach helped me to find my psychoanalytic position in relation to working with transgender young people, which presented me with an ethical challenge. I also discuss the ethics of conversion therapy to further illustrate the process and merits of systematic ethical analysis. These examples serve as reminders of the importance of prioritizing the patient's personal values to mitigate the dangers of a normative ideology guiding the analytic process whilst retaining the integrity of our own understandings and values, which may differ from the patient's. Finally, I critically examine the 'interpretation of the transference' as an example of the importance of questioning what drives adherence to the analytic techniques that we privilege.

Teaching ethics in a psychoanalytic training all too readily becomes token. Rules and codes of ethics cannot protect the patient against the operation of the therapist's unconscious. Protection can be increased, however, through *how* we teach ethics, which is the focus of Chapter 8 where I set out a possible curriculum with specified readings. This chapter concludes the book with a discussion of the training implications embedded in the arguments put forward in earlier chapters. The quality of a training, I suggest, is largely determined by what we are encouraged to question in ourselves, in our method and in our institutions. I propose that any training that takes ethics seriously should provide much more than the study of the code of ethics, or a handful of seminars on sexual boundary violations or on confidentiality. Without doubt these are very important areas that require reflection, but ethics cannot be reduced to 'topics' that we can tick off as 'covered' as part of seminars taken once during training, and often not until the midpoint in training. Such an approach reinforces parochial and technical conceptions of professional life that do not guarantee ethical practice. If rules and standards have a place in our work, they can only be meaningful if they are implemented responsively, that is they need to be considered with respect to the patient's needs at a given point in time. This requires *ongoing* critical consideration of the patient's and therapist's respective internal and external contexts. Supervision, of course, can and does contribute to this. It is necessary but, in my view, not sufficient.

Aristotle recognized that both moral and non-moral skills require training and practice. This is not about achieving perfection—an impossibility—but about striving towards doing our very best. One of the primary functions of a psychoanalytic training should be to help candidates develop a space in their mind that acts as an inner applied ethicist in relation to the therapist's own practice, that is the ethical chóros. Every intervention that we make or fail to make in a single session with a patient has ethical implications: we must always balance the risks and benefits of what we do for the patient at a given moment and recognize the responsibility that we bear towards him. A training should also embed values that enable candidates to feel able to consider and debate the moral life that dwells in the institution in which they train and of the structures of the society in which they practice. Engagement at this broader systemic level is vital to the reform that our psychoanalytic institutions need with respect to questions of power and diversity of various kinds. This requires teaching in ethics to be integrated into the very fabric of trainings throughout.

A note of gratitude

As I hope will be clear by now, my primary goal is to articulate a framework for thinking about the ethics of our work and the ethical dilemmas we face as clinicians. To this end, I draw on many inspiring voices within psychoanalysis, bioethics, and moral philosophy. Some of the ideas I present are therefore not wholly new—for example, others have written eloquently about the inherent asymmetry in the analytic relationship or more broadly about the centrality of ethics to psychoanalytic practice and I will introduce you to their work in the pages to come. I owe much to the psychoanalytic colleagues who have straddled the two disciplines long before I applied myself to their integration.

My studies in ethics taught me many things. I had the privilege to contemplate mind stretching questions. What makes death bad? Is it morally preferable to improve the lives of specific people or of future people? Does an algorithm have agency? The content of these debates was not directly relevant to my clinical work, but the *process* of working through ethical questions was. It helped me to be more disciplined in challenging cherished beliefs by looking at different sides of an argument in a thorough and balanced manner. It reminded me that we cannot simply believe that option/interpretation A is better than option/interpretation B: we need to have *good reasons* for why we opt for A or B. The different debates we covered brought home to me that for many of the ethical dilemmas that we face, there is no absolute right or wrong answer, only better (i.e. more logically coherent, truthful, other-focused) or worse arguments[1] for and against our decisions. Most importantly, studying ethics encouraged me to keep firmly in mind, time and again, that facts and values are

---

[1] I am using the term 'argument' in its philosophical sense, meaning a set of reasons that justify a position.

not dichotomous but entangled, and ultimately that ethics is about people, not arguments.

During this time, one book stood out for me—it would be on my list of 'desert island' books. It is a book by the moral philosopher Janet Radcliffe-Richards (2012) about the ethics of organ transplants: *Careless Thought Costs Lives*. The controversial subject it tackles is irrelevant to the present text. However, the book's brilliance, and the essence of applied ethics, is that it urges us to be alert to how 'careless thought costs lives', that is how we think about an issue has practical far-reaching implications for those affected by the issue, whatever that may be. How we think about our work, about our aims, about what we hate as much as what we love about being a psychoanalytic clinician, tangibly, and ethically matters.

A note about terminology

For readability, I have opted to use the pronoun 'she' for the therapist and 'he' for the patient unless I am specifically referring to individuals who identify as 'they'. In so doing, I am not wishing to undermine transgender therapists or patients who use the pronoun 'they'.

In referring to the relationship between patient and therapist, I refer to the 'analytic relationship' and not the 'therapeutic relationship' to denote that it is specifically psychoanalytic therapy/psychoanalysis under discussion and not psychotherapy generally.

I use the generic term 'therapist' to encompass psychoanalytic psychotherapists and psychoanalysts too. If I am making a sharp distinction between the two, I will signal this. I am only discussing (psycho)analytic psychotherapy and psychoanalysis and my arguments are articulated in relation to the specificities of this particular modality of therapy.

Throughout the text, I frequently use the modal verbs 'must' or 'ought'. Such verbs indicate, amongst other things, obligation. I use such verbs intentionally because I am addressing the aspirations—the 'must'/'ought'—for our practice and for our discipline more broadly. This is not an unconscious moral bias in my thinking—it is a very explicit intention.

Where I have used clinical session material, I have reused material published previously (with consent) or else I have opted for fictional composite cases that provide an illustrative narrative about relevant dynamics without any session detail.

I have a penchant for etymology. . . . I am all too aware that this is not to everyone's taste and can seem precious. Nevertheless, I hope that some of the insights that it is possible to derive when one reaches back into the roots of words might offset some of the initial reservations.

Finally, and at the risk of this sounding like a pre-emptive strike to deflect possible criticism, I want to explain my decision to use at times extensive quotations from other sources. My decision to do so, which is not characteristic of all my writing, is that in this text I want to have a conversation and bring to life the ideas that have inspired and informed me. Sometimes, allowing the original sources to speak for themselves, struck me as more fitting and potentially more helpful than my synthesis of the ideas I have digested, especially if this text is used for training purposes.

1

The Unbearable Silence
of Responsibility

To a large extent the danger posed by the first meeting [with a patient] arises from the prospect of a fresh encounter with one's own inner world and the internal world of another person. It is always dangerous business to stir up the depths of the unconscious mind. This anxiety is regularly misrecognized by therapists early in practice. It is treated as if it were a fear that the patient will leave treatment; in fact, the therapist is afraid that the patient will stay.

(Ogden, 1992: 227–228)

Unless we are to say that psychoanalytic function takes place in a conflict-free autonomous zone of the ego, we have to allow for the problems involved not only in digesting the patient's projections, but also in assimilating our own responses so that they can be subjected to scrutiny. The analyst, like the patient, desires to eliminate discomfort as well as to communicate and share experience; ordinary human reactions.

(Brenman-Pick, 1985: 157)

The myth of the analytic situation

The first and most fundamental principle that we need to grasp when we begin training as a psychoanalytic therapist—the one from which flow the normative foundations of a potentially helpful analytic relationship—is that psychotherapy unfolds in an interaction between two people who bring to bear their respective conscious and unconscious minds on the process.[1] The second important principle is that the analytic encounter implicates two flawed and fallible subjectivities. These self-evident yet profound facts are obscured by the projections we typically make onto the respective positions of 'patient' and of 'therapist'. Muriel Dimen reminds us that 'there exists in psychoanalysis a deep structure that aligns analyst and patient in two separate columns: knower/known, wise/ignorant, powerful/needy, and so on' (2021: 70). Heinrich Racker (1957) understood this only too well when he described the 'myth of the analytic situation', namely the belief that psychotherapy is an interaction between a sick person (the patient) and a healthy one (the therapist): '. . . The truth is that . . ., in both . . . the ego is under pressure from the id, the superego, and the external world' (Racker, 1957: 307).[2] In other words, each party brings to the analytic encounter a unique mix of developmental history, cultural influences, longings, passions, prejudices, and fears, only some of which will be consciously recognized.

In an ironic twist, it appears that as psychoanalytic clinicians we display a remarkable ambivalence towards the core tenet that guides our work: '. . . the irreducible features of the unconscious' (Harris, 2007: 363). An uncomfortable implication of the very notion of the Freudian unconscious, as Lacan observes in his seminal work on ethics, is that '. . . the analyst is fully aware that he cannot know what he is doing in psychoanalysis. Part of this action remains hidden even from him' (Lacan, 1992: 291). This means that the therapist can strive to act responsibly but may yet be subject to unconscious regressive pulls that undermine ethical behaviour. Indeed, the process of psychoanalysis is, at its core, a process of 'accepting responsibility

---

[1] The title of this section—'the unbearable silence of responsibility'—is taken from Zygmunt Bauman (1993: 78).

[2] It is not only the therapist who is vulnerable to sustaining this split. The patient, too, may need to locate the therapist in the 'healthy' category for his own defensive reasons. However, I am focusing here only on the implications for the analytic process of this split when it is more or less unconsciously subscribed to by the therapist.

for one's own unconscious' (Lear, 2003: 7), and this applies to both parties. However, much as we might aspire to be 'partners in thought' (Stern, 2010), we are not *equal* partners when it comes to responsibility for what transpires in the analytic setting.

The so-called 'myth of the analytic situation', which fosters forgetting or minimizing recognition that the therapist is also flawed and fallible, in my view, accounts for some of the ethical transgressions or errors that we are all susceptible to making in the course of our work. It is not a question of 'if' but of 'when' and of 'how' we transgress or 'get things wrong'. What matters is how we respond to the impact that our actions have on the patient and take responsibility. Being responsible does not necessarily mean one has *caused* the 'bad' thing to happen, whatever that might be in an analytic dyad, though there will be times when this is indeed the case. It means that when things go wrong, the therapist must step up (i.e. take responsibility) and ensure that what has happened can be thought about non-defensively, truthfully, and fairly.

The challenge we face is how to maintain a *horizontal relationship* with the patient. By this I mean, a lateral, structurally similar relationship of equals based on the dimensions of respect for autonomy, veracity, and justice. This horizontal relationship of equals is established and protected through 'generous imaginings' (Scarry, 1998: 50) that root us in a respect for the patient's otherness. Maintaining horizontality requires a consistent effort at balancing recognition of similarity and respect for difference (Benjamin, 1998). The horizontal relationship is inevitably in danger of being subverted by the uniqueness of the needs and defences generated by the meeting of two unconscious as well as conscious minds. This can tip the relationship into a vertical one.

There are two types of verticality, and it is important to distinguish them. I will discuss *malignant verticality* shortly, but first let's consider what I am calling *benign verticality*, which is unavoidable because although patient and therapist are equals in terms of fundamental rights as human beings, the therapy is *for* the patient and provided by the therapist. These roles are not equal: they carry different expectations, degrees of power, and responsibility. Only one party (the therapist) has (a) *asymmetrical responsibility* for the setting of therapy and for what unfolds within this setting and (b) has *positive duties* towards the patient (i.e. what a therapist should and should not do). We ignore the unavoidable power differential in the analytic relationship at our peril and to the potential detriment of our patients. Even the most egalitarian, well-meaning therapist cannot circumvent the asymmetry of the analytic relationship. The best we can do is to recognize it and not abuse it.

The psychoanalytic promise

Ethics, as I use the term throughout this book, refers to how we think about and manage our responsibility for the patient. I want to be clear about how I use the word *responsibility*. If we return to the etymological roots of the word, from the Latin *spondere* meaning 'to give assurance, to promise', the person who is responsible is fundamentally one who *makes a promise*. I suggest that the 'psychoanalytic promise' involves availing oneself to be made 'use' of by the patient in the service of helping him with his mind, within the agreed boundaries of the analytic setting,[3] and not impinging on this 'use' with our needs or desires. For me, supporting the patient's shift from *object relating*, where the object is needed but not completely perceived as other, to *object usage*, where there is a realization that the other is outside one's boundaries and is separate (Winnicott, 1969), is one form of ethical work central to the analytic telos that I will set out in more detail in Chapter 3. Our ethical responsibility lies in protecting the patient's safe passage from the necessity of relating to us as an internal object to using us as an object to discover himself as a separate subject, which is how I understand the distinctive contribution of an analytic process compared to other types of psychotherapy.

---

[3] It is important to emphasize the latter because by its very nature the analytic relationship will mobilize intense longings in both parties. Just as the therapist needs to respect the boundaries, so does the patient: the boundaries of the analytic relationship (e.g. set time, absence of physical contact; restricted access to the therapist outside of session times) anchor it in reality; this can be experienced as cruel or depriving by the patient.

The parameters of the therapist's responsibility are defined by the duties or obligations inherent to the role of therapist.[4] Because the patient is seeking psychoanalytic therapy or psychoanalysis specifically, he has a right to expect a particular kind of psychoanalytic care and understanding that considers the operation of an unconscious mind. The psychoanalytic promise is a pledge to attempt to decipher the unconscious as it manifests within the patient and between patient and therapist. This pledge requires that the therapist be willing to recognize that her unconscious is always operative, and can potentially impact on the patient, and be committed to examining and taking responsibility for this impact.

In *How to Do Things with Words*, the linguist and philosopher, J. L. Austin (1975) includes the speech-act of 'the promise' under the category of the so-called 'commissive'—a category that involves a commitment by speakers to certain courses of action. The status of the promise is therefore importantly temporal, casting the speaker into a future time when she will deliver on what was promised. I suggest that the promise, in the context of psychotherapy, is the overarching frame of the work: we are working with the patient because we have made a promise to undertake a very particular type of work over a period of time. The ethics of psychoanalytic work are in the service of holding out on this promise with due attention to whether the interventions we make respect the patient's autonomy, do not harm him, maximize benefit for him, are fair and truthful. This does not necessarily mean that we can always help the patient at all or in line with his hopes and expectations, but that we strive to do so to the best of our abilities, for as long as we have good reasons to believe that we are helpful,[5] all things considered. The temporal dimension of the promise thus roots us in the prospective nature of ethics (i.e.

---

[4] It goes without saying, that there are the objective obligations as well as the unconscious fantasized or wished for obligations. For example, the patient may well wish for unrestricted access to his therapist and may feel that the therapist is not discharging her obligations if she fails to respond to a request for help outside of session times. Unless this was agreed as part of the analytic setting, this would represent a wished for 'obligation' that is therefore to be understood and interpreted in the context of the transference.

[5] We might, of course, disagree about whether we should even be aiming to be 'helpful' as this aim is not unanimously considered appropriate to the analytic endeavour—see, for example, Robert Caper's (1999) discussion of this issue.

what we should do and must avoid doing in future in order to not injure others). Elaine Scarry (1998) refers to this as 'prospective morality' noting how much harder it is to practice than 'retrospective morality' (1998: 43) when we judge actions that have already taken place. Focusing on the future, on the promise and how we might break it, implicates us more directly as moral agents.

It has often been suggested that the analytic situation reinstates the asymmetry of the infant–adult relationship where the infant exists in a radical dependency on others for its survival (see, for example, Chetrit-Vatine, 2014; Scarfone, 2014). Recognizing the vulnerability that necessarily attends subjectivity—insofar as the subject is given over to others from the start—has ethical implications. The concept of vulnerability has become central to feminist interventions in ethics, not least in the 'ethics of care' (Gilligan, 1982).[6] These approaches underscore how the condition of universal vulnerability has a normative force. They place special emphasis on mutual interdependence and emotional responsiveness. Indeed, one way to think about ethics is that it is fundamentally concerned with how relationships are best nurtured and how they are always at risk of being destroyed—a concern that is shared with psychoanalysis. Therefore, in a very fundamental sense, and because of this risk, psychoanalysis needs ethics given the centrality of the analytic relationship to the process and outcome of therapy for the patient.

I foreground the therapist's asymmetrical responsibility because its recognition is central to ethical practice—a point that has been eloquently made by others, not least Viviane Chetrit-Vatine (2014) and Mitchell Wilson (2012, 2013, 2020) whose writings I highly recommend. Our work demands that we understand the nature of this responsibility, its requirements, and its emotional costs (to the therapist). Returning now to what I call *malignant verticality*, this concerns how the analytic relationship can be destroyed or undermined or, if you prefer, how the original promise is broken. It refers to the perversion of the axiomatic asymmetrical responsibility, that is when the therapist's power is deployed to meet the therapist's

---

[6] See Glossary for definition.

conscious and unconscious needs and/or desires. Here, it is power that dominates the relational field, not care. When this happens, we foreclose the possibility for the patient to make 'use' of us as an object. Transgressions and other ethical breaches invariably undermine the patient's ability to 'use' us. This is because an act of transgression or breach typically results from the therapist relating to the patient as an object in her own internal world and not as a separate subject. Jessica Benjamin's (2004) contributions are especially important in this respect as she recognizes the work required of the therapist to monitor the inevitable slippage between recognition of the other as separate and as an internal object, that is belonging to our internal world and projected onto the other.

The therapist's ethical labour: Managing love, desire, and hate for the patient

Because the analytic relationship is so central to the analytic process and outcome, our attention must squarely focus on the demands placed on the therapist if she is to put her 'self' in the service of the patient's psychic well-being. This is a very particular kind of *ethical labour*. I refer to it as an ethical labour because I have in mind a type of work and accountability that implicates the therapist at an unavoidably personal level. This is an exacting process. It requires that we bear being loved, desired, and hated by the patient, and in turn to manage *responsibly* our love, desire, and hate for the patient. In practice this means that we are responsible for mentalizing our own feelings towards the patient.

Let me now explain what I mean by this. Loving and sexual feelings towards our patients are normal and need to be responsibly managed. I am sure that we will have all, most likely, worked with a patient who, were it not for the circumstances in which we meet them (i.e. someone who turns to us for professional help), might have been someone with whom we would have otherwise potentially enjoyed a friendship or felt sexually attracted to. At the very least, we may feel a lot of affection for the patient and in some cases we may even feel love and erotic desire towards the patient. These are all normal, expectable reactions to our patients. The challenge is how we manage the attachment and sexual feelings that the analytic relationship can also mobilize so as to not impinge on the patient, especially when his needs for correspondence of such feelings match the therapist's thus opening up a path towards potential unethical enactments.

When I refer to desire, I do not only mean the therapist's erotic desire. I also have in mind what Wilson (2013) has helpfully articulated as our more 'experience near derivatives' (2013: 440) of what we desire from the patient, such as the 'intentions, aims and values that motivate our actions' (Wilson, 2013: 440) and that have consequence for the patient. As Wilson observes in his work in this area, which deserves careful reading, 'It is obvious that analysts want things in and from their work and want things from their patients' (Wilson, 2013: 446). There is an unsurprising resistance to registering the 'Procrustean bed of the analyst's desire' (Gruenberg, 1995: 434). As if reckoning with the inevitable intrusions of our desire were not enough, we also have to contend with our hatred towards the patient. This hatred may result from a thwarted longing for care and attention in the therapist, potentially setting up a competition for scarce resources where the patient is perceived to be receiving what the therapist feels she is not getting, or the therapist may experience the patient's rejection of her efforts to help as a kind of deprivation, which may trigger the therapist's rage (Racker, 1968). It is important to specify that when I refer to hatred of the patient, I have in mind hatred of his dependency or contempt or of how he may at times need to make us feel inadequate or guilty or excluded, not that we hate him in any absolute sense.

The ubiquity of the regressive pulls towards love and hate that we are subject to during our daily practice, I suggest, should be where our learning begins when we embark on training. The challenge in our work lies precisely because of the pressure exerted by both impulses. Understanding this ubiquity is central to ethical practice and should be prioritized in our curricula and what we are encouraged to think about upfront, as I will argue in Chapter 8. Yet, it was only some years into my analytic training that I recall being set as reading Winnicott's (1949) classic paper 'Hate in the Countertransference'. At the time, I mused: why did we not start with *this* paper? Winnicott's recognition of why our work can be so challenging is essential reading at the start of training. Given the level of abstinence required of us in our work, it should not surprise us that we can hate the patient who is felt to deprive us or criticizes us. The ethical therapist is not the one who does not experience this tension: it is the one who recognizes it because she expects it and can then mentalize it. As Sarah Ackerman notes:

> The ethical conduct that analysis requires invites the analyst to deceive herself; she is asked to aspire to a position in which everything she does is what is best for the patient, an assumption that denies her basic human nature. Only by holding an awareness of this conflict can the analyst fulfill her ethical role. (2020: 567)

Winnicott, more than any other, helps us to understand that the therapist, like the mother, can legitimately hate the patient, some of the time. He stresses two key points. First, that acknowledgement of this hatred enables us to sustain our capacity to be with the patient. In other words, it is essential to know about our hatred or else we cannot do our work. Winnicott's notion of an 'objective countertransference' is relevant here. He was referring to those aspects of the therapist's feelings about the patient that derive not from pathology in the therapist or in the patient, but instead reflect the range of 'normal', to-be-expected feelings such as fear or hate and that coexist with love and concern for the patient. It is important that we recognize this objective countertransference.

The second crucial point that Winnicott articulates is that the patient needs the therapist to recognize her hatred for him in order to enable the patient to experience and express his own hatred. He emphasized that this experience is developmentally necessary. Being a kind, compassionate therapist who cannot register her own hateful feelings towards the patient, Winnicott suggests, may thus constrain the patient's exploration of his own hatred. Let me go further: we cannot underestimate the developmental importance of allowing the patient to hate us and to recognize when we hate the patient. This is because there exists a close connection between hate and autonomy: hate that can be mentalized supports the delineation of a sense of self and that is the first step towards autonomy.

Recognition of the inevitable interactional pressures bearing on the analytic dyad sensitizes us to the psychic roadblocks that both patient and therapist create and that may derail the psychoanalytic promise. Neville Symington (1983) alerts us to the internal prohibitions brought to bear on the analytic relationship by both parties who can join to create a superordinate system that preserves the status quo, undermining development. By contrast, he believed that an 'act of freedom', as he put it, breaks apart the unity of the system and opens opportunities for new relational configurations. The opposite of an act of freedom is what I consider to be the all-too-common unconscious *narcissistic pacts* that can transpire between patient and therapist, for example the therapist's pathological accommodation to the patient's needs and demands in order to not incite the patient's anger or hatred. Narcissistic pacts set the conditions for unethical behaviour (see Chapter 5). It is down to us to increase the margin of ethical choice by gaining insight into the 'blatant deals', which as Erikson cautioned, '... not only virtue and vice, but also the ethical and the moral, are attempting to make within us and right in front of us' (1976: 413).

We need to work against the pull of our narcissism. Narcissistic pacts are more likely when we fail to recognize the tensions between love and hate for the patient or if we neglect Wilson's reminder that the therapist always wants something from the patient. Slavin and Kriegman (1998) propose that conflict in the analytic relationship derives from the inherently diverging interests (identities and needs) of therapist and patient that result in what they term 'conflicts of interests'. In their view, these are an ever-present part of the landscape of the analytic relationship. Rather than framing this as pathological, but still surely requiring a special effort on the part of the therapist to do no harm, they normalize this interactional reality:

In myriad forms and innumerable deceptive ways, our subjective worlds and our interests will conflict with those of our patients . . . . Woven into the most loving and cooperative motives (over and above the influence of professional roles) every individual organizes—really must organize—his or her subjective world to communicate and promote his or her own interests. (Slavin and Kriegman, 1998: 252)

The inevitability of this clash of interests, they argue, is the quotidian backdrop to our work that, I suggest, we do well to anticipate if we are to keep our psychoanalytic promise. The ethicality of our decisions about how to intervene with our patients is determined by our willingness to assume responsibility for the unconscious investments embedded in our decisions, to own our desires and our hatred and to understand their unique coordinates. It involves questioning who we are and taking a hard look at our own histories, individual and collective. Ethics requires a commitment to the truth of our responsibility for the analytic relationship we create and inhabit with the patient.

Not unlike the adult on a flight during an emergency landing who should first pull down their own oxygen mask so that they can then assist the child, the therapist must prioritize understanding and managing her own mind before she can assist the patient with his. By this I do not mean that it is therefore essential for us to have our own therapy or analysis. I take this for granted. But the experience of personal therapy during training is only a foundation. The kind of self-knowledge that is relevant to psychoanalytic work is an ongoing process that requires self-monitoring and ethical scrutiny of our own mind and intentionality, in every session, with every patient, hence why ours is indeed an 'impossible profession', as Freud (1937) cautioned.[7] It is worth reminding ourselves of Freud's observations:

Among the factors which influence the prospects of analytic treatment and add to its difficulties in the same manner as the resistances, must be reckoned not only the nature of the patient's ego but *the individuality*

---

[7] I will argue, in Chapter 3, that we have a duty of self-knowledge.

of the analyst. It cannot be disputed that analysts . . . have not invariably come up to the standard of psychical normality to which they wish to educate their patients. . . . Analysts are people who have learnt to practice a particular art; alongside of this, they may be allowed to be human beings like anyone else. After all, nobody maintains that a physician is incapable of treating internal diseases if his own internal organs are not sound. (1937: 247–249, my italics)

Revisiting countertransference

Psychoanalysis provides, par excellence, the key technical concept that should assist the therapist in understanding and managing her intense emotional reactions to the patient: the concept of countertransference, which has been variously defined. Freud's (1909) first mention of the term is in his written response to Jung about what we now recognize as a sexual boundary violation: the affair Jung had with his then patient, Sabina Spielrein. Freud's advice to Jung was unambiguous: he should strive 'to dominate' his countertransference. However, despite being clear about what Jung should do, it is evident from Freud's response to Jung that Spielrein, the patient, was framed as a 'difficult' patient. Freud displayed in his writing about her a 'cold objectification' (Kahane, 2018: 459) framing the source of the problem as Spielrein's, not Jung's (Pinsky, 2017; Wilson, 2013). Unfortunately, there are still abundant clinical discussions of patients—especially female patients—that similarly frame the problem in this manner, reminding us of the pernicious ongoing impact of misogyny within our own discipline (Chamberlain, 2022).

In a discussion about enactments, Wilson (2020) argues that what we often attribute to the patient is in fact a '*misattribution*'. He draws attention to a dangerous bias in a significant proportion of the literature on countertransference where the interactional process is presented as a one-way street: the patient does something to the therapist who may or may not then be drawn into responding because of what the patient did. This is an ethical slippery slope: where does responsibility lie when things go wrong? Despite Freud's reluctance to attribute any responsibility to Jung for the origin of his erotic feelings, he was nevertheless clear that it was Jung's responsibility to manage the desire once activated in him.

When the concept of countertransference was first elaborated in Freud's time, therapists regarded their emotional reactions to the patient as manifestations of their own 'blind spots'. In 1912, Freud stated that the therapist should behave:

> . . . as a surgeon who puts aside all his own feelings, including that of human sympathy and concentrates his mind on one single purpose, that of performing the operation as skilfully as possible. (1912: 115)

The metaphor of a surgeon who performs a clean-cut incision without the interference of her feelings profoundly shaped the analytic persona that therapists internalized for many years, supported by the armoury of the rules of abstinence, anonymity, and neutrality—the classical psychoanalytic ethical triumvirate. However, Paula Heimann's (1950) work drew attention to a different version of countertransference, one that favoured the therapist's emotional response to her patient as a technical tool, not a hindrance. This viewpoint has profoundly influenced current contemporary practice. Bion's (1963) steer to resist the temptation of 'memory and desire'[8] in the clinical situation in favour of reliance upon our emotional experience as the only 'facts' available to us, signposts the contemporary emphasis on countertransference as a privileged source of knowledge about the mind of the patient. This position implies that we have access, through our own emotional reactions, to knowledge about the patient's state of mind, without this knowledge requiring explicit communication through the spoken word.

From Kleinian and many object-relational perspectives, countertransference includes all the therapist's reactions to the patient,

---

[8] Bion argued that memory was misleading because it was subject to the distortion by unconscious processes and desire (to cure) interfered with the capacity to observe and understand the patient.

no matter what their source, allowing for greater tolerance of the therapist's subjectivity. However, this understanding is not at all the same as an intersubjective approach to the therapist's subjectivity. In Kleinian approaches, the therapist's task is to understand, through the countertransference, who she comes to represent for the patient at any given point in time whilst simultaneously remaining connected with who the therapist is when divested of these projections. This, as we all know, is easier said than practiced because, as Dunn observes:

> . . . the therapist's perceptions of the patient's psychic reality are also constructed through, and distorted by, the lens of unconscious fantasy. It is untenable to assume that the therapist is an objective observer, simply mirroring the patient's transference. (1995: 725)

It is indeed difficult to see how it would be possible to *reliably* separate out our emotional reactions as a response to the patient's unconscious communication from our own so-called neurotic reactions. As Kernberg reminds us:

> The therapist's conscious and unconscious reactions to the patient in the treatment situation are reactions to the patient's reality as well as to his transference, and also to the therapist's own reality needs as well as to his neurotic needs. This approach also implies that those emotional reactions are intimately fused. (1965: 49)

Although the concept of countertransference gained momentum especially within the Kleinian school, in fact the note of caution about its potential misuse also originates within that same school, not least from Melanie Klein. Spillius (2007) notes that Klein urged the therapist to examine herself first, before framing the patient as the source of the feeling in the therapist:

> I have never found that the countertransference has helped me to understand my patient better. If I may put it like this, I have found that it helped me to understand myself better. (Klein quoted in Spillius, 2007: 78)

These concerns have led some therapists to caution that the countertransference understood in an extended manner may expose the patient to harm because all the therapist's reactions emerge from her personal and subjective position, yet the concept encourages framing the therapist's action as '. . . a re-action, an action "again," following the action of the patient' (Wilson, 2013: 437). As such, the concept may be used to dilute the therapist's agency.

During any analytic relationship, we will project onto our patients and experience temporary partial identification with them, but our commitment is to relate to them as separate and not be confused with ourselves. This requires vigilant monitoring of our own projections because the interaction that evolves between the therapist and the patient is determined by unconscious forces operating in both. Inspired, yes, but the concept of countertransference is therefore also problematic because it is predicated on the assumption that the therapist can distinguish what feelings belong to her from those that the patient projects into her. Acknowledging this challenge is nothing new. However, by linking it closely to ethics, I want to revisit this with a renewed emphasis by reclaiming the value of Freud's original definition of countertransference as something that requires our constant attention and consideration of it as an ever-present *ethical risk*, rather than primarily as a technical tool that advances our work. We nod theoretically to this risk but our emphasis in clinical discussions and publications is mostly illustrative of the added value of the countertransference. Unless we are careful to qualify the use of the concept, working through in the countertransference as a technique reinforces a basic assumption that is inimical to ethical practice: the assumption of the patient's transparency and of our own transparency to ourselves.

Using psychoanalytic knowledge responsibly

More than other psychoanalytic theories, the intersubjective and relational schools have challenged the classical positivist view of the therapist's objectivity. The critique of the general project of the

Enlightenment and its knowledge claims, found a clear voice in Owen Renik's (1993) original paper, which called into question the reductionist premises of mainstream psychoanalysis. He claimed that the therapist's work is determined in significant part by her personal psychology, and he argued for a systematic reconceptualization of analytic technique that presumed the therapist's 'irreducible subjectivity'. Both intersubjective and relational therapists uphold that we cannot approach clinical material as if it were an entity that exists in the patient's mind, conceptually isolated from the relational matrix from which it emerges. As approaches influenced by post-modern thinking, they also highlight contextuality and perspective over universal proclamations that apply to all situations regardless of historical contingency, culture, or gender. Through these different emphases, they call for a more inclusive and egalitarian dialogue about the nature of the analytic relationship, displacing the notion of the therapist's epistemic authority.

The notion of the therapist's subjectivity, and the attendant limitations imposed on the therapist's claim to objectivity, is a conceptual currency that has now crossed the ocean and contributes to theoretical discussions across different schools of psychoanalysis (beyond North American ones) around the question of so-called 'localization' (Ringstrom, 1998: 214), that is who is responsible for what in the analytic dyad. The work of therapy has thus been reframed as the exploration and interpretation of the patient's subjectivity within a context that acknowledges that the analytic dialogue and process will reflect, and be constituted from, the mutual and inevitable unconscious emotional interactions between therapist and patient with the subjectivity of each contributing to the form and content of the dialogue that emerges.[9] To argue otherwise, in any polarized fashion, is difficult to defend. Recognition of the subtly complex nature of the mutual influence of therapist and patient on each other is essential to ethical practice because it is impossible to argue that the therapist,

---

[9] Ogden (1994) refers to intersubjective reality as the 'analytic third'. He contends that the therapist's responses are never fully individual events. Rather, the meaning of the therapist's reactions is always a newly created reality by virtue of the original, never-to-be-repeated interactions of the specific analytic couple.

as a person, has no impact, or that the therapist, by virtue of her own training analysis, is beyond being tripped over by her unconscious. In other words, what transpires in the consulting room is inevitably influenced by the therapist's own psychology. In this spirit, Slavin and Kriegman (1998) describe the 'psychic undertow' that characterizes all intimate relationships:

> In an overarching, often unconscious way, each [party] attempts to use the other, to pull the other into his or her subjective world, and to resist the pull, the undertow, in the opposite direction. Simultaneously, though, each needs to 'use' the other to construct his or her own identity and thus wants—must want—to take in aspects of the other's subjectivity. Each tries to redefine the other in his or her own terms (and both to accept and to resist redefinition in the terms of the other). We call these universal relational tensions an undertow because they operate inexorably beneath whatever crashing of waves and ebbing and flowing of behaviours catch our attention on the surface. (1998: 249–250)

The core of psychoanalytic inquiry during an analytic process is therefore not directed at the mind of the patient alone even though it is exclusively *in the service of* the patient's mind and his psychic development.

By now you might understandably think that along with my ethical turn I have also taken an 'intersubjective turn' in my psychoanalytic identity. This is not the case, and it is important for me to clarify this upfront to avoid confusion. Even though I have found it stimulating and essential when thinking about ethics to learn from intersubjective and relational colleagues and their assumption of bi-directionality, I remain strongly identified with an object relation tradition at the level of my understanding of psychic development and of analytic technique. What do I mean by this? I mean that for me, the two-person model of intersubjectivity is highly relevant but it does not cancel out the force of intrapsychic reality or the value of also focusing on the latter within an analytic process. Moreover, although there is ethical merit in the position that highlights the risks associated with the 'broader' concept of countertransference (Wilson, 2020), the concerns I also share about this, are not in the service of making the case against any broadening of the concept: the challenge is *how* we make use of it and what is required of us to deploy this technique ethically. Irma Brenman-Pick's (1985) now classic paper, 'Working Through in the Countertransference', stands out as an excellent example of this. Although the word 'ethics' does not feature in her paper, I suggest that she demonstrates the essence of applied ethics in a psychoanalytic session through her carefully attuned tracking of the countertransference, her humility, and willingness to question herself, her recognition of the complexity of the dynamics between patient and therapist, and her ongoing concern for what is best for the patient. Brenman-Pick helps us to appreciate how we can responsibly use the countertransference as the basis for developing our understanding about the patient even if such 'knowledge' can only be partial. In the chapters to come, I outline more specifically how a principled approach can support us in this task.

The inter-subjectivists, unlike the relationists, regard even a two-person psychology as problematic because they understand it to still embody '. . . an atomistic, isolated-mind philosophy in that two separated mental entities . . . are seen to bump into each other' (Stolorow et al., 2002: 95).

Problems inhere within such a pure intersubjective position. One danger is that it can feed into a view of the analytic relationship as functionally symmetrical, which in turn distances the therapist from awareness of the inevitable asymmetry, as I suggested earlier, that can expose the patient to risk. Without recourse to the respective contributions in mental life of an internal *and* external world, of reality *and* phantasy, it becomes even more difficult to discern who is impacting whom and to reflect on the nature of the conflicts arising both within and between therapist and patient. This is as problematic, in my view, as the position that privileges the countertransference in its broader sense. Acknowledgement of the 'psychic undertow', and of the provisional and partial nature of our judgements and interpretations, is not an argument against the possibility of holding—at least some of the time—a more objective position (than the patient) about what unfolds in the analytic process and using this to formulate a clinical opinion.

By de-emphasizing the contribution of the patient's intrapsychic functioning and foregrounding relational interaction, a purely intersubjective position begs other important questions, such as the role of the patient's developmental history that informs interpersonal and affective patterns established *prior* to engaging with the therapist. We all start a therapeutic journey primed in highly specific ways by our prior experiences; the transference is operative before the first session even though the actual meeting will most likely shape it in particular ways because of the bidirectional nature of all human exchanges. These prior expectations and experiences constitute a partial truth about the patient as an individual who brings something pre-existent and unique to the analytic encounter and to a therapist who is trained to decipher his personal psychic signature. Our training must count for something or else why train or why seek a therapist if we don't expect that she has something additional to offer—I will return to this point later.

We must recognize the difficulty of disentangling the influence of the other in self-knowledge and of deciphering how we impact on each other. However, this does not mean that we cannot strive to make any objective assessment of our patients. It simply means that we must carefully attend to the investments we make in this knowledge and qualify accordingly how we share this knowledge with the patient and use it. What matters then to the ethics of the analytic encounter, is our *relationship to knowledge*, which is most appropriately conceptualized as evolving and requires openness to being challenged and to revision. The value of an intersubjective perspective, I suggest, resides in providing a corrective to the risks inherent to analytic arrogance, which we are all vulnerable to, reminding us that the ethical priority is the cultivation and exercise of *epistemic humility*. This should not be confused with the relativism of the postmodern turn, which carries its own risks, not least when it privileges the personal and individual and downgrades any discourse that strives to distinguish between internal and external reality and make some observations about 'objective' reality. Epistemological privileging of the patient's narrative is not the basis for a truly collaborative analytic dialogue—*respect* for the patient's narrative is. Respect provides a safe context for the exploration of differences in understanding with the shared goal of helping the patient with the problems that brought him into therapy in the first place.

If we return to the central question of 'who is impacting whom?', it may then be more accurate to claim that our attempt to answer it is inevitably hedged by our blind spots, hence partial. We are invariably speaking about an approximation of what we believe to be going on in the patient's mind *and* in our mind. Therefore, ethical analysis is essential to practice because we are forever precariously balanced on the tightrope between 'my needs' and 'your needs', between 'my understanding' and 'your understanding'. We need a space in our minds—what I term the *ethical chóros* (see next section)—in which to critically question what we do and why we do it so that we steer the best course for the patient who has entrusted us with his mind, but without abdicating ours in the process. Difference in all its guises, and respectful engagement with it, is a stimulus to thought. Ethics is partly about protecting the conditions in which difference can safely contribute to the patient's psychic development.

Developing the *ethical chóros*

In 1799, the eighth Astronomer Royal at Greenwich, Neville Maskelyne, came across an interesting finding. He identified discrepancies of approximately 0.8 of a second between his own observations of the transit times of stars across a hairline, measured by counting the ticks of a pendulum clock, and those of his assistant. On this basis, he boldly fired the assistant: as far as Maskelyne could understand at the time, his assistant was imprecise and doing a bad job. It was only some twenty years later, in 1820, that the German astronomer and mathematician Friedrich Wilhelm Bessel followed up Maskelyne's report with his own discovery. Bessel observed that even skilled astronomers vary consistently in the transit times that they report. Based on this finding, Bessel introduced the 'personal equation' for calibrating these individual differences in what later came to be called 'reaction time'. Thanks to Bessel's work we now recognize that any measurement requires correction of a person's characteristic reaction time: we obtain different results because of individual difference, that is we each see the world differently.

I suggest that each therapist has the analytic version of the *personal equation*. We each understand the same behaviour in a patient or take it up the transference in subtly different ways because of the inherent individual bias when it comes to perception. This should not surprise us given the existence of an unconscious mind that is highly idiosyncratic in its perception and experience of reality. We also each introduce unique potential 'triggers' to the analytic mix by virtue of being who we are with our characterological dispositions, our unique 'givens' (e.g. our sex, a visible disability) and how we inhabit our bodies and the physical space we create in our consulting rooms. Paul Denis also explicitly uses the term 'personal equation' in the following passage:

> The analyst should take into account the fact that his personal equation is not ipso facto neutral for everyone, and should anticipate, in a 'responsible and asymmetrical way', the effects of the setting that he proposes at the heart of which his character has a central place. (2011: 80)

I do not know whether Denis is informed by the origins of the term that I shared above for context, but his passage suggests that he is using the term specifically to denote the impact that the therapist's individuality—her 'givens'—has on the setting. For example, he refers to the physical attractiveness of the therapist that may be especially affecting for some patients and not others. He rightly emphasizes that the therapist's personal equation '. . . is not . . . neutral for everyone' (Denis, 2011). In practice, it may mean that the therapist, say by virtue of a given about her physical appearance (e.g. having a particular type of physical frame), presents the patient with an undeniably personal aspect of her being that is emotionally arousing for a particular patient. It is indeed helpful to conceptualize the body of the therapist as an integral embodied part of the analytic setting that impacts differentially on patients (Lemma, 2014, 2019). An aspect of our ethical responsibility thus involves recognition and management of our personal equation, in the specific sense intended by Denis. However, I am using the term in a second sense too.

When I refer to the therapist's personal equation, I also use it to denote very specifically the therapist's inevitable *unconscious listening biases*, due to our unique developmental experiences, our cultural milieu and our theoretical allegiances. All these influences implicitly impose an idiosyncratic listening frame on the analytic encounter (see Chapter 4). Even though nowadays most therapists acknowledge theoretically that there is a degree of personal influence due to the therapist's individuality, I have suggested that we do not focus on this enough *in practice.* My impression is that this is routinely acknowledged but just as quickly set aside when we prioritize an intrapsychic focus as we listen to the patient. Consequently, the potential usefulness of our recognition of the personal equation for examining the unfolding of a session is undermined, with a specific implication for how we think about the ethics of our work. However, as Jane Kite points out, ethical practice requires us to attend to this:

> Significantly, most of our character (as distinct from our characteristic style) is unconscious at any given moment, yet also decisive for the action of the analysis. Another way to put this might be that the analyst as a person (as opposed to a role) is psychically and materially the central organizing fact of any analysis, and in this way takes on an unimaginable responsibility with each new analysis. (2016: 1159)

In a very insightful and moving paper about work with patients whose former therapists have committed a boundary violation, Dianne Elise teases out the emotional demand imposed on the patient when it comes to recognizing that the therapist's own character may be unhelpfully impinging on the work—even when there is no gross ethical violation at play. I quote Elise at length because her clear articulation deserves it:

An analyst's character/countertransference problems are not easy for a patient to identify *with confidence*. Feelings of uncertainty abound: 'Did I know something was 'off'—yes, no?' The analyst has not committed a boundary violation in any overt, clearly recognizable sense. Instead, the analyst's narcissistic rigidities and subtle lapses in integrity contribute to a treatment stalemated or broken off, with a patient left traumatized. Such character difficulties in the clinician can include inappropriate ways of handling a patient that antagonize or humiliate or otherwise undermine the patient's state of mind. An overinvestment in adherence to a particular theoretical model and wedded technical approach can result in abuses of interpretive power, with interpretations functioning as accusations. Clinician defensiveness can be cleverly disguised by lines of interpretation that, although they may be accurate, obscure an entrenched countertransference stance that persistently does not recognize or admit the clinician's contribution to an impasse. Although patients can and certainly do play their part in impasses, it takes two to *tangle*. (Elise, 2015: 559, italics in original)

Each party also brings to the analytic encounter different *value systems*. Meissner encapsulates very well the inextricable nature of 'being a therapist' from the therapist's personal values:

the analyst himself cannot be divorced from his ethical and moral values, nor from the value-system in which they inhere. That value-system is part and parcel of his personality structure, his character, and there is no way that it can be eliminated from his participation in the analytic process. It is an essential dimension of the reality of his person, and thus plays an integral role in the interaction, transferential and otherwise, that unfolds between himself and the patient. Consequently, I would conclude that the value-free immunization concocted by analytic theorists with regard to the analytic process cannot be maintained. (1994: 459–460)

In one sense, of course, we can never fully know the nature of our personal equation—of what might skew our understanding, of how our bodies communicate far more than we can fully consciously grasp, of the personal vulnerabilities that can be triggered in the analytic exchange and then impact on it—given that we can never fully know our own unconscious. Even so, acknowledging that there are limits to this knowledge, as I suggested earlier, is not an argument against the possibility of any knowledge. We can and should take responsibility for striving to know as much as we can about how we impact our patients. Part of our moral duty of care—what I refer to as the *tripartite duty of care*—to the patient requires that we strive to be:

(a) Cognizant that the ethical relation is asymmetrical and that we consequently carry asymmetrical responsibility for safeguarding the boundaries that are constituent of an analytic process.
(b) Open to recognizing, and to taking responsibility for, the impact on us, and therefore on the analytic relationship, that results from the ethical demand inherent to our work because the patient is a separate agent whose needs will conflict (at times) with our needs.
(c) Committed to monitoring and responsibly managing the impact of our personal equation on the patient.

This tripartite duty of care captures the essence of an ethical attitude to psychoanalytic work that, at its best, functions like a setting in the therapist's mind towards the patient (Wiener, 2001). The nature of our responsibility as therapists means that we must be receptive to the anxiety that flows from it, resist its disavowal, and find ways of managing it. One of the primary functions of a psychoanalytic training should be to help therapists develop what I term the *ethical chóros*,[10] that is a space in the therapist's mind that acts as an inner applied ethicist in relation to the therapist's own practice. The *ethical chóros* denotes a *principled* internal space that regulates our practice through supporting self-questioning in relation to our work with the patient and the obligations we have towards him, the most

---

[10] From the Greek, χῶρος meaning a clearly defined space/environment—it is a dwelling space (which is quite different from a 'chorus' (χορός), a band of singers and dancers, even though it is phonetically similar).

fundamental of which is that we must first create and safeguard in our mind a dwelling space for the patient and his singularity. This requires us to critically reflect on our personal equation and how this impacts selectively, depending on the patient.

The *ethical chóros* is the space in our mind for self-reckoning in relation to our work. This principled space ought to be the constant background, much like we expect the analytic attitude to be.[11] Let me go further. The development of the analytic attitude—that cornerstone of analytic work cutting across diverse conceptualizations of psychoanalysis—can only be articulated in relation to the *ethical chóros*. In fact, it does not conceptually make sense to distinguish them because the analytic attitude is rooted in ethics (see also Scarfone, 2017), but for our purposes I am distinguishing the *ethical chóros* to make explicit this core component of the analytic attitude.

The *ethical chóros* denotes an inner space of ethical reflection that can be supported through a consideration of the core ethical principles that I will introduce in Chapters 2 and 3 but reaches beyond these. Ethical practice relies on an *ongoing* commitment to a process of ethical self-scrutiny mindful that this can never result in a perfect self-awareness reliably affording the therapist a privileged position from which to understand the mind of the patient. The existence of the unconscious, and the operation of defences, reminds us that self-reflection is always hedged by failure. As Judith Butler eloquently puts it, it is an 'open-ended and unsatisfiable attempt to "return" to a self from a situation of being foreign to oneself' (2005: 129). Again, this is not to say that giving an account of how we understand the patient is impossible or has no value, but rather, that its possibility is limited in various ways, such that we always and necessarily fail to give a complete account.

The *ethical chóros* conceived of as a principled space that internally regulates our work needs to be distinguished from superego

---

[11] The analytic attitude, as I define it here, refers to the therapist's state of mind (i.e. her intentional state, that is, her beliefs, desires, feelings) in relation to the patient and to the work of psychoanalysis (i.e. receptivity to the unconscious and to the unfolding of the transference).

moralism as a guiding structure for practice. The latter pays short-term narcissistic dividends for the therapist when she lives up to its exacting demands and sustains temporarily a view of herself as somehow 'superior', but it fails to protect the patient. Instead, the *ethical chóros*, when it is functioning well, is rooted in the recognition of the inevitability of imperfection, hence of errors. It is not about pointing the finger at ourselves and saying 'you are bad'; it is about drawing our attention to how we do get things wrong at times and how we can 'do better' through supporting self-questioning in relation to our work.

Let me be clear, in referring to errors or flaws, I am not wishing to diminish the gravity of what can transpire between a therapist and patient as merely 'an error'. A therapist who has a sexual relationship with a patient gravely harms the patient and this is an ethical and potentially legal matter. However, such flagrant transgressions are fortunately the minority. It is the more quotidian errors or transgressions, and the less arousing ones for the profession and the public, that escape notice and yet can also perpetrate harms. The *ethical chóros* is the space we need to cultivate in our mind because it helps us to reflect on and regulate our practice in relation to *all* possible harms (see Chapter 5). This formulation chimes (for me) with Scarfone's (2017) emphasis on the *personal* ethical core of the practitioner:

> The idea is that psychoanalysis is such a unique form of practice that its ethics is not some moral superstructure, not something added to its Epistemology (or its Ontology), but rather that it precedes, is inseparable from and regulates the epistemological aspects of our practice. In plain English: our ethical stance is what allows (or impedes) central psychoanalytic facts to be brought into daylight. (2017: 394–395)

In the psychoanalytic literature there are several important elaborations of the notion of a 'third space' from which one can reflect on oneself. I will not review them all here but focus instead briefly on the Kleinian view as exemplified in Ron Britton's (2004) work and Jessica Benjamin's (2009) notion of 'thirdness'. I select these because they are most helpful to me in clarifying what I mean when I refer to the *ethical chóros*.

In his classic contribution, Britton (2004) linked the working through of the oedipal triangle to the development of the capacity to make use of what he called 'triangular space' which, in turn, paves the way for the establishment of a third position from which we can be observers and be observed. In this elaboration, the third is an oedipal construct and supports an internal observing function. At first glance, the intersubjective position that Benjamin (2009) refers to as 'thirdness' appears to share much in common with Britton's position. However, it is different in significant respects. In fact, her ideas are best conceived as elaborated in contrast to Britton's ideas (and those of other Kleinian colleagues), specifically her focus on building a 'shared third' with the patient. For Benjamin, thirdness requires both the therapist and the patient to surrender in the service of creating a transitional space where they can develop a sense of connectedness to each other while accepting each other's separateness and difference. She proposes the notion of the 'moral third or the third in the one' to denote the capacity to 'maintain internal awareness, to sustain the tension of difference' (Benjamin, 2009: 13) between the therapist's own subjectivity and needs and those of the patient. This enables the emergence of an experience of the interaction as 'something beyond' them as separate subjects. It is this 'something beyond' that is a 'third position'. Importantly therefore, the third is primarily an intersubjective *co-creation*, that stands as a desirable alternative to the asymmetrical complementarity of 'doer and done to', as she puts it.[12]

The *ethical chóros* shares features in common with Britton's self-observing position and with Benjamin's notion of the moral third, but it cannot be simply equated with either of them. I draw on a space metaphor—the chóros—to capture the mental space necessary for the internal ethical work the therapist needs to undertake

---

[12] Clinically, the concept of a co-created intersubjective thirdness helps to elucidate the breakdown into the twoness of complementarity in impasses and enactments and suggests how recognition is restored through engagement with the contribution we make to this complementarity.

so as to support the creation of the symbolic space of thirdness with the patient that Benjamin describes. I conceptualize the chóros as an inner space in which we reposition ourselves internally so that we can then return to the patient with a different perspective on what has happened, and may still be happening, between us and patient. This requires tolerating an experience of 'isolation' that comes from reckoning with our responsibility for the patient. We have to bear this alone, which is what I understand Bion to mean when he refers to the 'essential' 'sense of isolation within the intimate relationship of analysis' (1963: 15) and what Zygmunt Bauman evokes when he refers to the 'silence of responsibility' (1993: 78). The *ethical chóros* is thus best conceived as an essential part of the therapist's internal setting, which rests on the capacity for self-observation that Britton outlines but has very specific functions. I am therefore not describing an intersubjective process that could be understood as a transitional space co-created with the patient. Rather, I am referring to an intra-personal space that helps the therapist to monitor how her personal equation or her 'idols' can impinge on the patient and may thus impede thirdness, as Benjamin understands it.

Evidently there are some overlaps between the three concepts (i.e. Britton's, Benjamin's and my own), but there are two important differences. First, unlike the other two concepts that are more encompassing, I am specifying (a) a distinct feature of the therapist's internal setting with very clear *functions* in the service of supporting ethical practice and (b) the *processes* that unfold within this mental space, namely self-reflexivity and self-reflection. Being *self-reflexive* refers to how the therapist strives to critically examine her interactions via introspection as they occur in the moment with the patient. By contrast, in the *self-reflective* mode the therapist reflects post-hoc on various elements (verbal, nonverbal, feelings, and thoughts). The two perspectives, namely the in-the-moment and the post-hoc, interact and inform each other challenging and updating the therapist's *ethical chóros* and contributing to the consolidation of the ethical attitude, that is, our vision of what ought to be, and what is possible, in relation to each patient. The *ethical chóros* is thus the place for both self-reflexivity and self-reflection. Because it is an essential constituent of the therapist's internal setting, the *ethical chóros* needs to be developed during training and sustained beyond it since it provides the ethical dimension of the analytic attitude.

A second difference between the three concepts concerns their respective degrees of specification. A limitation of the notion of a third as an observer position, as Britton conceives it, or of Benjamin's thirdness, is that they can be abstract 'space' or 'position' metaphors. They are deeply evocative and useful for that reason. However, for a space metaphor to be of *practical* use to therapists, especially early on during training, it benefits from a further degree of specification so that the therapist can identify what she is trying to do when in that 'space' and can access key concepts that provide some conceptual scaffolding. Therefore, as I will elaborate in later chapters, I ground the *ethical chóros* in basic ethical principles (which I reinterpret within a psychoanalytic frame) that can be described and clearly referred to. This has implications for training, as I will later discuss in Chapter 8.

Key psychoanalytic contributions about ethics highlight the way that ethical codes cannot capture the complexity of the ethical task we face (e.g. Ackerman, 2020; Levin, 2010). For example, Ackerman emphasizes a 'moment-to-moment approach' to ethics (2020: 571), reminding us that we cannot apply rules to the analytic process in a general way. Universal and general ethical rules are useful guides but our reliance on them can conceal or distort the nature of the ethical demand specific to our work because they obfuscate the key ethical question, which concerns specificity, that is *for whom* we are required to act in a particular way. However, whilst this is a necessary caution, I suggest that we still need access to a more explicit ethical framework, not of codes but of 'principles in action'. Especially early on in training, when we face ethical dilemmas or attempt to evaluate the ethics of our work, we may feel too disoriented without recourse to conceptual touchpoints that can assist us in the 'moment-to-moment' ethical wrangles.

Accountability is deontological in nature, in other words related to rules and to what is allowed, but when we are discussing the ethical task in the 'moment-to-moment' we are concerned with how we can most effectively support the therapist's capacity to 'think well' about how to do the right thing—this is not about rules, but about how we think about our work. To think well, we are assisted by conceptual scaffolding. Of course, any framework or structure that organizes and guides thoughts and actions within a reasonably well-defined domain needs to be dynamic and constantly subject to critique and open to revision, from both inside and outside the system. Ethical frameworks are no different in this respect; that hardly makes them invalid or useless. Nor does the application of a particular framework to a given horizon of problems or questions preclude the concurrent application of one or more other approaches to the same set of problems, when that might yield further insights or potential solutions.

The focus I am placing on self-reflexivity and self-reflection about ethical issues has not been traditionally a central preoccupation in our discipline, even though the North American literature, in particular, now attests to a much stronger and resilient interest in the importance of conceptualizing ethics. However, many trainings in the UK, for example, still only have relatively few seminars on ethics. Perhaps this remains the case because, as Hester Solomon observed in one of the few notable British (Jungian) contributions to this subject, '. . . many analysts feel as if thinking about ethical issues is an unwelcome disruption or intrusion into the real analytical task' (2004: 250). That said, I hope that you will persevere, turn the page, and consider how ethical principles are not an intrusion into our 'real work', but what make our work possible.

2
Bioethical Principles

And finally, we must not forget that the analytic relationship is based on a love of truth—that is, on a recognition of reality—and that it precludes any kind of sham or deceit.
—(Freud, 1937: 248)

The 'ethical turn' in many disciplines, including more latterly in psychoanalysis too, gained momentum in the late 1990s, prompted by a return to questions of obligation, respect, and recognition. In this chapter, I set out the Four Principles model (Beauchamp and Childress, 2013) as it exists within bioethics before addressing its more specific psychoanalytic framing and application in Chapter 3. It is important as a profession that we agree to act on principles that we can view as principles *for all*. This is what allows us to then articulate an account of ethical requirements specific to psychoanalytic practice in addition to those principles consistent with any professional 'caring' role.

The Four Principles model is based on four common, basic prima facie[1] moral commitments, namely respect for autonomy, beneficence, non-maleficence, and justice. Although it does not typically feature in psychoanalytic writings, I suggest that this model offers a foundational moral analytical framework and a common moral language that is well suited to analytic practice, with some additional specifications. My aim in this chapter is not to critique the model, but merely to outline it for the clinician-reader who is not

---

[1] Prima facie obligations are those that we ought to perform, in and of themselves.

acquainted with it, drawing attention to the complexities it raises but also highlighting how the principles invite helpful questioning of our clinical practice.

The Four Principles approach

One of the main objectives of morality is to minimize pain and distress and to prevent or limit the disadvantage(s) of those who are suffering. Ethical principles are in the service of furthering these aims. Ethics begins with the question: what morally ought we to do? It then provides general rules of duties or obligations[2] as guides to action. Within the Western philosophical tradition, ethics involves formulating, justifying, and recommending certain principles of conduct applicable to all rational beings. In each case, I am required to think of myself and others as subject to the same universal moral rules, whatever the differences that may exist between us, which are deemed arbitrary and irrelevant from a moral point of view.

Ethics supplies us with a moral map that we can use for thinking through more systematically the clinical dilemmas that we encounter and for evaluating the ethics of our clinical work. *Bioethics* refers specifically to the study of moral issues pertaining to the fields of medical treatment, clinical research, and overall patient care. It aims to establish what physicians, mental health professionals, and researchers should and should not do, their so-called positive duties. Tom Beauchamp's and James Childress' (2013) Four Principles framework is the dominant approach in bioethics today. As an approach, it is generically referred to as *principlism*. Instead of evaluating clinical decisions by means of a specific full-scale moral theory, principlism is intentionally consistent with a variety of general moral theories (e.g. utilitarianism, Kantian deontology, and virtue ethics).[3] The four principles it promotes do not therefore depend on a specific moral theory for their content and justification.

---

[2] I will use the terms 'duties' and 'obligations' interchangeably.
[3] See Glossary for definitions.

This is one of the strengths of principlism because it operates within a set of moral norms that are generally accepted as reasonable by people subscribing to a wide variety of moral traditions. It brings together many of the most plausible elements of different ethical theories into a clear and pragmatic framework:

> the four principles should also be thought of as the four moral nucleotides that constitute moral DNA—capable, alone or in combination, of explaining and justifying all the substantive and universalisable moral norms of health care ethics. (Gillon, 2003: 308)

The potential risks of ethical relativism and ethical moralism respectively are well recognized in discussions about moral norms. Principlism offers two advantages in this respect. First, it provides a basis for a very widely accepted set of ethical commitments, which can help us avoid ethical relativism. Second, the recognition that there are morally legitimate differences in how we interpret or prioritize them given the specifics of each case, introduces sufficient flexibility to avoid so-called moral absolutism (Gillon, 2003).

At the heart of Beauchamp and Childress's account are the principles of beneficence, non-maleficence, respect for autonomy, and justice. All four principles, and the more specific moral norms that stem from them, generate prima facie obligations that are not absolute and thus permit exceptions. The principles are equal in significance: no individual principle trumps another, and efforts must be made to avoid violation of any one of them. However, any one of the principles can be potentially overridden by a weightier principle. If one principle is overridden, for example if we prioritize third-party safety by arranging a patient's compulsory admission to hospital because he *may* pose a risk to others at the cost of respecting the patient's autonomy, the effect of the violation of the other principle (in this example, autonomy) should be minimized.

Although proponents of deontological theory would argue that there are universal ethical principles that apply to all situations, most clinical dilemmas cannot be resolved by applying the principles in a rote manner or have only one 'right' response. For example, when working with an adult patient who reports suicidal ideation and who does not want to be admitted to hospital, there is no undisputed universal rule for handling the dilemma between respecting the patient's declared (i.e. consciously stated) wishes and acting to ensure the patient's physical safety thereby potentially undermining the patient's autonomy.

Let's now look at each principle in more detail.

Non-maleficence

Non-maleficence, or not inflicting harm, is often expressed as *primum non nocere* (first, do no harm). Typically attributed to Hippocrates, and often invoked in medical and psychotherapy ethics, it was the French pathologist and clinician Auguste François Chomel (1788–1858) who first introduced it as a medical axiom as part of his oral teaching in Paris (Herranz, 2002). The much-invoked principle is nevertheless challenging to implement: defining what constitutes a harm is a complex matter. This is both because harm is a subjective experience and because some harms may be justifiable in specific contexts:

> A harm is a thwarting, defeating, or setting back of some party but a harmful action is not always a wrong or unjustified one. (Beauchamp and Childress, 2013: 153)

For example, a therapist who breaches an ethical code, may have to endure sanctions that impact her livelihood (i.e. cause her harm), but this does not mean that the punishment (a harmful action in terms of the negative impact this would have on the therapist) is therefore wrong.

Although there are some general norms of human needs, benefits, and harms, people vary in their individual perceptions and evaluations of these. What I consider to be a benefit, or a harm may be highly idiosyncratic. Jehovah's Witnesses attitudes to blood transfusions are a common illustration of this variability. Moreover, we need to draw a distinction between collateral or short-term harms in the service of longer-term goals and harms that cannot be justified by recourse to more overarching ends. In the context of psychotherapy, an interpretation may temporarily destabilize a patient and be experienced by him as harmful because it sets him back (e.g. he may feel unable to work for several days following the session) but we could argue that such temporary setbacks, along with the subjective experience of harm, are justified by the longer-term benefits (e.g. the patient's depressive state improves). This is often the case in medicine where the 'cure' can sometimes be as bad as the illness that prompts it.

As in medical treatments, it may be more accurate therefore to say that as therapists we work to ensure that the benefits of our interventions outweigh the risks. This relies on an assessment of the relative balance of risks and benefits of any given intervention. In this sense, *do no harm* may be too simplistic as a guide to ethical practice given that some collateral harms are inevitable in many treatment interventions. This is especially relevant to the psychoanalytic endeavour that works to challenge psychic structures that are in place to protect the patient from thoughts and feelings that are felt to be subjectively harmful and yet, such a defensive structure may also be very costly to the individual (Steiner, 1993). However, relinquishing defensive structures may temporarily be experienced by the patient as a worse state. Indeed, such potential though not certain risks should be discussed with a patient. Not doing so deprives the patient of an opportunity to give informed consent and this, in turn, undermines autonomy (see following points).

Thus, even to attempt to benefit people with as little harm as possible, requires exploration of not only what the patient regards as a harm but also the least harmful of the available options. Moreover, even if the patient agrees that one available intervention would be more beneficial than another, he may simply wish to reject the beneficial intervention on other equally important (to them) grounds. This may be because of an idiosyncratic basis of assessment of harm. For example, and to return to the case of a Jehovah's Witness, consider the belief that a blood transfusion will lead to eternal damnation, or consider the patient who views his homosexual orientation as the source of harm to his family and requests help to become heterosexual.

Beneficence

The principle of beneficence exhorts us to positive actions to help the patient to further his interests. It concerns the *obligation to help*. It is worth emphasizing that, in distinction to non-maleficence, the language here is one of positive requirements, of the moral importance of doing good to others. The principle calls therefore not just for avoiding harm but also to benefit the patient and to promote his welfare. More specifically, doing good is thought of as doing what is best for the patient. This principle is critically important because it urges us to consider individual circumstances and values and to keep in mind that what is good for one patient may not necessarily be good for another and may not concord with what the therapist thinks is good for the patient. Values are idiosyncratic and subjective, hence decisions about what is best can only be considered on an individual basis.

One of the biggest shifts in healthcare generally, and which pertains to psychotherapy too, is that the principle of beneficence, which traditionally was invoked to justify paternalism, is nowadays trumped by autonomy: the patient decides what is best for him. Beneficence is usually considered to rely on an objective view of what would be best for the patient whereas respect for autonomy identifies what the patient subjectively considers to be in his best interests. There is therefore an inevitable tension between these two principles: a vulnerable patient may, because of an internal and/or external situation, make treatment decisions that are arguably not in his best interests. An obligation to act in the best interests of a patient may become paramount when working with individuals whose capacity for autonomy is diminished because of lack of understanding, extreme distress, serious disturbance, or other significant personal constraints.

The very idea of 'best interests' is complex. As a concept, 'best interests' is linked to the notion of *well-being*. This refers to how well a person's life is going for that person, that is a person's well-being is what is 'good for' them (Crisp, 2021). Well-being is a kind of value, sometimes called *prudential value*, to be distinguished from, for example, aesthetic value or moral value.[4] The standard view is that well-being is an agent-relative value (i.e. it gives reasons to the agent whose well-being it is). Hence, if something increases my subjective sense of well-being, then I have reason to desire it and pursue it, and similarly for you and your well-being. In each case, the reason-giving fact for the agent is that his 'good' would be enhanced or at least not diminished.

In medicine, not least because treatment options have increased and expose the patient to complex choices, it is more standard practice to explicitly consider patient values to identify the best option. This requires the doctor to engage with the patient in a normative and values focused dialogue, as well as exchange of facts, to identify what would best promote this patient's well-being in a specified context. Moreover, nowadays medical interventions are no longer restricted to offering treatments that will cure a medical or psychological condition. The aims of treatment are not bound by the narrower conception of health as the absence of disease but extend to include interventions that will enhance the psychological and/or social well-being of the person (Savulescu et al., 2011).

There is no general agreement about constitutes well-being as reflected in the different accounts of well-being (hedonistic, desire-satisfaction, objective list theories)[5] (Fletcher, 2016). Theories of well-being are often categorized as being either subjective or objective. Subjectivism states that nothing can intrinsically enhance the quality of an individual's life unless the person desires or endorses that thing. Objective theories do not include such a requirement. Hence, something may be deemed good for an individual even in

---

[4] The emphasis is on something being 'good for' a given person and it is therefore not an indicator that the life in question is necessarily a morally good one.

[5] See Glossary for definitions.

the absence of a relevant pro-attitude, for example, the importance of having good relationships in one's life. More recently, a composite *welfarist view* of well-being has been proposed which includes hedonistic, desire fulfilment and objective elements (Savulescu et al., 2011). This latter conceptualization is relevant to the ethics of psychoanalytic work because it challenges us to consider that well-being depends on the values and interests of the individual, placing at its centre pluralism about value (i.e. the view that more than one thing makes up well-being). This approach to well-being most clearly exposes the tension between the authority invested in medical and psychological 'expertise' about what makes a life go well and the individual's right to choose what he considers to be in his best interests. It gives considerable weight to the individual's own desires and evaluations of his interests.

The welfarist approach proposes that what is of intrinsic value is well-being itself. When something reduces someone's well-being, the harm this reduction perpetrates is considered intrinsically bad. This approach has been applied as a challenging alternative to how we conceptualize mental health problems. Roache and Savulescu (2018), for example, propose replacing the term 'mental disorder' with 'psychological disadvantage', linking this to the importance of well-being where 'promoting well-being differs between patients, depending as it does on each patient's values and interests' (Roache and Savulescu, 2018: 249):

> According to this approach, a person has a mental disability if they have some stable psychological trait (or set of such traits) that makes it likely that their life will get worse, in terms of their own well-being, in the social and environmental context they inhabit . . . . Because what counts as a mental disability depends on individual circumstances, a trait could count as a disability for one person but not for another. (Roache and Savulescu, 2018: 249)

By foregrounding well-being as a central organizing principle, the welfarist model allows us to approach 'health' in terms of the ability of the individual to create a way of living that fits his idiosyncratic disposition, values, and needs rather than in terms of a rigidly fixed norm. This emphasis is relevant to the question of values and the role they play in the analytic relationship with regards to beneficence. Therapist and patient may have different views on what constitutes a problem. Even framing something as a 'problem' reveals that there is variation with respect to how a problem is evaluated (i.e. felt to be good or bad) by the patient. To recognize an evaluative element is important because it helps us to clarify its contribution to the conceptual framework we deploy. It also foregrounds the importance of giving due weight to patient values in determining *whether* to intervene, and if we do, how to best promote the patient's welfare given the patient's values and aspirations. To this, I suggest that we add, that assisting a patient to identify his values is enhanced when we factor in the operation of an unconscious mind given that our values may be unconscious or unarticulated (Lemma and Savulescu, 2021)—I will return to this point later.

The shift in prioritizing patient values because they are central to well-being, invites us to consider whether an intervention is, all things considered, better for a person if the benefits that enhance that person's overall well-being outweigh the harms. To enable meaningful consent to any treatment, we therefore need to engage with the patient to understand his values and particular life circumstances, relationships, and position in society and to think through how the intervention can support those values and aims and at what cost (physical and/or psychological).

Inevitably there will be cases where an individual's values conflict, or sometimes we might question whether the patient's values should change. For example, if working with a patient who gains gratification from duping others and for whom such behaviour is egosyntonic, we must consider whether the aim of working with such a patient would be to help him to take stock of the violence he perpetrates against others through duping them even though the patient himself may not perceive anything 'wrong' with this way of relating. I will not dwell here on the complexities that such cases raise in relation to how we understand our role and what we mean by 'being neutral', but we will return to some of these themes in Chapter 3.

However, even though it is not a focus of this book to debate whether the purpose of psychoanalysis should be to help the patient not only understand his desires and motivations but also what he *should* do and help him to do it, I suggest that grappling with this question in ourselves is central to ethical practice. I will illustrate further the complexities introduced by considerations of values and well-being in Chapter 7.

Autonomy

You will notice that, comparatively speaking, I devote more space to a discussion of autonomy than the other principles. This is because, as I will also return to in Chapter 3, respect for a person's autonomy is axiomatic to ethical practice and, in my view, supporting the development of the patient's autonomy is a central aim of analytic work. For our psychoanalytic purposes, my last statement requires some qualification, but first we need to unpack the concept of autonomy as it stands in bioethics.

In ethics, autonomy refers to self-governance, privacy, individual choice, liberty to follow one's own will, and being one's own person. The expression of and respect for autonomy revolves around the individual: its conditions require capacities internal to the person, whilst recognition of autonomy demands non-interference with a person's subjective values, beliefs, and preferences. For an action to be autonomous, there should be clarity that the person choosing is acting intentionally, with understanding, and be free of controls either from external sources or by internal states that '. . . rob the person of self-directedness' (Beauchamp and Childress, 2013: 138).

The normative criteria of autonomy are neutral towards the actual content of one's desires, commitments, and values. Different choices, values, and conceptions of the good life are warranted respect, regardless of their potentially dubious value to others. This value neutral stance contributes to the *individualist focus* in many discussions about autonomy. The philosopher and economist, John Stuart Mill concentrated his efforts on the importance of protecting liberty and respecting autonomy, which he referred to as 'individuality'. He argued that because we have 'privileged access' into who we are and what matters to us, we are the best arbiters of how to exercise our 'individuality' even if this results in what turn out to be poor choices (for us):

> If a person possesses any tolerable amount of common sense and experience, his own mode of laying out his existence is the best, not because it is the best in itself, but because it is his own mode. (Mill, 1910: 115)

The individualist focus of autonomy traditionally conceived as a matter of independence from others and their preferences, has not gone without challenge. Critics question the primary focus on the individual and argue instead for a broader concept of *relational autonomy*—one shaped by social relationships and complex determinants such as gender, ethnicity, and culture. In these critiques, autonomy is understood as embedded within, rather than opposing and transcending, the reality of human vulnerability and dependency, which may very well preclude our full mastery of external circumstances. We are all socially situated amid complex relations with other people and are bound by interpersonal frameworks that exert significant influence upon our lives. These facts, the critics contend, have significant implications for autonomy.

One such critic, Marina Oshana (2014), has proposed a 'social-relational' account of autonomy as a condition of human being, one that is largely constituted by the presence or absence of a person's relations with other people, which she argues, is what determines whether the person can develop and retain the influence and authority required for self-determination. For her, personal autonomy is thus constitutively and intrinsically social and relational. Camillia Kong's (2017) equally important work helpfully traces how, in mainstream bioethics, autonomy remains a feature of the individual will. A consequence of this is that the criteria for autonomy simply require that our decisions accord with our own preferences, values, and desires. Like Oshana, Kong argues that this focus neglects crucial relational, social factors that bear on the development and exercise of autonomy. She underlines what she regards as the contemporary idealization of subjective mastery and self-reliance implicit in some models of autonomy, which reinforces a view that autonomy cannot coexist with dependency. As will be apparent, both Oshana's and Kong's critiques are very consistent with a psychoanalytic position. Judith Butler (2005), too, has foregrounded our shared vulnerability as defining of the human condition and argues that it is precisely this shared condition that motivates a call to ethics. As Catherine Mills explains in her study of Butler's work, our vulnerability as humans is indicative of the way that each of us is 'given over' to others from the start:

> This common condition of being given over entails that the subject is never able to attain the moral ideal of a self-directed, rationally motiv-ated, and wholly self-knowing agent. But rather than stymieing efforts towards ethics, this 'failure' is ultimately generative of ethics, insofar as one recognises these limits as the shared predicament of oneself and all others. (2022: 42)

Relational accounts of autonomy[6] thus challenge us on two fronts. First, they encourage us to think in a more nuanced manner whereby, for example, the capacity to seek assistance and support from others can itself be an important indicator of autonomy. In other words, having a realistic notion of our constraints, limitations, as well as possibilities is crucial to autonomy. It permits, as David Black puts it, for 'an ethical claim' (2020: 1002) rooted in our intersubjective nature, to have authority over the claims of 'sovereign autonomy' (David Black, 2020: 1002). Second, these accounts invite us to criti-cally assess the socially constituted content of our self-narratives and how these can promote or discourage autonomy. A central question

---

[6] It's worth noting that these accounts are also highly relevant to how we think about 'iden-tity politics', which has raised a plethora of ethical questions that currently impact on clinical practice (see, e.g. Chapter 7 where I share my experience of navigating the ethics of working with transgender young people). In a trenchant discussion about identity politics, David Pilgrim discerns '. . . a general vulnerability in all forms of identity politics, where individual assertion for freedom (autonomy) and unchallengeable self-definition might also reflect nar-cissism and even solipsism ("it's all about me")' (2022: 69).

concerns the extent to which features inside or outside of the individual (i.e. broader societal and relational factors) bear on autonomy. In the accounts where autonomy is thought to revolve around the internal structure of the individual, Kong (2017) proposes that autonomy is conceptualized as a type of 'competence'. By contrast, when external, relational forces are thought to affect autonomy, the assessment of autonomy reveals itself to be much more complex and nuanced. Relational approaches to autonomy thus focus on how intersubjective, social conditions shape and contribute causally to the development of autonomy and hence identity. Our personal developmental histories and socialization are indeed central variables. Our bodies, our ways of perceiving and thinking, are all socially inscribed. This is a key point. It reminds us of the ethical necessity of respecting the importance of taking ownership of our own volitions and desires whilst not neglecting consideration of their originating source,[7] which may undermine the authenticity of our consciously stated wishes.

The so-called 'authentic self' is key to understanding autonomy: 'who' is deciding? How to locate the 'authentic' self nevertheless remains deeply controversial within philosophy and ethics because this immediately raises the question of the impact of an individual's social context on the very nature of the authentic self. Authenticity conditions are said to be met when we make decisions based on '. . . desires, goods, or values that are our own, validated through a reflective process of first-personal identification' (Kong, 2017: 57). If the desires, goods, or values that inform a given choice can withstand such reflective scrutiny, then a decision that needs to be taken is thought to express the authentic, governing self. However, as we know, in practice it is far from easy to establish which desires are authentic and what we may have identified with through projective processes. Consider the example of a patient with an eating disorder[8] who subjectively endorses the value of thinness and alternates this with bingeing: restricting her eating makes her feel better

---

[7] I would add here that we should not ignore their impact on others.
[8] See also Kong (2017) for a discussion of autonomy in relation to anorexia.

in herself whilst bingeing makes her feel very ashamed, but she refuses help with a 'problem' that she believes is only a problem for others. In family therapy sessions, it becomes clear that her mother also prizes thinness and controls what she eats, and that both mother and daughter inhabit a social and cultural milieu in which being thin is valued and where 'not being thin' is linked with body shaming. Despite the patient's conscious assertion that she is 'choosing' to be thin because she likes how it makes her feel about herself and does not care about what others think, we might question whether the value placed on thinness is discordant with autonomy given that such a value emerges out of family dynamics (the mother-daughter relationship) and a sufficiently oppressive social context (i.e. societal pressure on women to be thin), thus making this patient's choice *heteronomous*, that is, subject to a standard that appears to be hers but is actually derived from external sources.

It matters to some notions of autonomy—the notion I endorse in this book—whether our wishes and desires are the product, for example, of restrictive social norms, dysfunctional and coercive family systems, individual relationships, our own internal racist or homophobic ideas, or any kind of abusive internal object, as we would understand it through the psychoanalytic process of unconscious identification. If we agree that such influences are relevant, this implies that some form of self-knowledge and self-reflection is therefore required to determine what is true and non-alien to the self.

Making distinctions between internal and external factors bearing on autonomy poses further challenges. This is because external influences—such as the family system we are born into—are not just causally implicated in who we are. In many ways they shape and inform, and hence may limit or enhance (depending on our experiences) our ability to reflect on and understand ourselves. The causal link between socialization and the authentic self therefore cannot be so neatly delineated due to its impact on the development of personal identity. As Kong observes, such external influences may be '. . . so well integrated with our identity that where the "authentic self" begins, and the impact of socialization and of our relationships ends, is unclear' (2017: 66). Socialization runs very deeply, and numerous aspects of our external environment may restrict our agency, reminding us that autonomy is not an either/or scenario—in practice it is infinitely more complex.

Taken together, all the preceding considerations, informed by relational accounts of autonomy, make clear why there is a critical difference between the 'freedom to choose', which refers to executive control at a particular moment in time and in a given situation, and 'autonomy' which depends on the assessment of a whole way of living one's life. Moreover, perceived self-control over a very particular sphere in our life does not necessarily imply autonomy. This distinction is very important clinically. For example, some individuals who choose to modify the body through cosmetic surgery may well feel in control in the moment they decide to undergo surgery and consider this choice to exemplify the exercise of their self-determination (i.e. autonomy), but in some such cases, as the therapist, we might understand this as only creating the illusion of control of, and freedom from, an internal object unconsciously identified with a body part that is removed or reshaped (Lemma, 2010). This is not autonomy.

Acknowledging the machinations of the unconscious reminds us of the limits to autonomy. Does this mean therefore that autonomy is an illusory state forever subverted by the unconscious? This requires some qualification. Autonomy is not an 'all or nothing' state. To this extent claims about autonomy in relation to the unconscious are always relative. I am making the more modest claim here that '. . . exploration of unconscious drivers supports the *expansion* of the range of autonomous functioning, not that it makes us autonomous in an absolute sense' (Lemma and Savulescu, 2021: 6). This points to the need for a nuanced understanding of agency, such as the one articulated by Stephen Frosh:

Subjects are produced by and in power; that is, they are constituted by social forces that lie outside them, in the workings of the world. But subjects still have agency; their agentic status is what they are produced with, and it enables them to take hold of power and use it. This does not mean that they are freed from the external operations of power, but it does endow them with subjectivity, with a richness of imagination, if one

> wishes to think of it that way. It means that they engage with power and are not merely its dupes or its obedient and loyal 'subjects'. (2015: 383)

We have agency but the conditions in which we exercise our agency are not fully under our control or always accessible to us for reflection (i.e. we may be unaware of them).

Considerations of autonomy are directly relevant to the concept of *paternalism*. Paternalism refers to the interference of a state or an individual with another person against their will. Typically, a paternalistic stance is defended or motivated by a claim that the person interfered with will be better off protected from harm. Intuitively we would all recognize that there are benevolent and malevolent forms of influencing another person. The principles of beneficence and non-maleficence suggest that as therapists we need to be cognizant of our ability to influence the individuals with whom we work. Let's consider a therapist working with a female patient who discloses domestic abuse. Adherence to the principles of beneficence and non-maleficence might lead this therapist to encourage the patient to leave her abusive partner to promote her physical and psychological well-being. In such a case, any kind of interventionist stance—however subtle—would evidently be related to the therapist's own (presumably) anti-violence values and exposes a paternalistic stance: the therapist, well-intentioned, would be nevertheless, more or less explicitly, steering the patient towards a particular outcome.

Although many therapists often argue that therapy should exist in a value-free context and advocate neutrality as a central psychoanalytic value, others suggest that it is impossible for us to be value-free and neutral. In our role as a therapist, we need to consider how *our* values, even when our intentions are to help the patient, can lead us to take up a paternalistic stance that potentially infringes on the patient's autonomy. After all, we all explicitly or implicitly subscribe to a view of what constitutes healthy psychic functioning, and this invariably guides what we prioritize in our interventions:

> Whether goals of treatment are proposed or simply implied, psychoanalysts should ask for whom these good outcomes are so desirable, and

what unexamined social forces, unconscious investments, and neurotic compromises in the analyst are involved. (Kirshner, 2011: 1226)

An ever-present risk in analytic work, and thus a potential harm for the patient, is that the notions we espouse of health can unwittingly allow the re-entry of old-style paternalism and the imputation of desires and values at an unconscious level on the patient. We will return to the question of our values in Chapter 3. For now, suffice to say that if we don't acknowledge the impact of our values on our work, we are at greater risk of being paternalistic. This is because what is important to autonomy is that patients can choose an option which is ultimately less than the best, as we might conceive of it (e.g. Jehovah's Witnesses refusing life-saving blood transfusions).

Paternalism is often divided into *soft* and *hard*. In *soft* paternalism, the therapist acts on grounds of beneficence (and, at times, non-maleficence) when the patient is nonautonomous or substantially nonautonomous (e.g. cognitive dysfunction due to severe illness, depression, or drug addiction). Soft paternalism is complicated because of the difficulty in determining whether the patient was nonautonomous at the time of decision-making but is ethically defensible if the action is in concordance with what the therapist believes to be the patient's values. *Hard* paternalism is action by a therapist, intended to benefit a patient, but contrary to the voluntary decision of an autonomous patient who is fully informed and competent, and it is generally regarded as ethically indefensible.

In the clinical situation, more precisely, we need to consider whether paternalistic behaviour that interferes with a person's autonomy is all things considered wrong, and so impermissible, or only *pro tanto*[9] wrong, and so possibly permissible, or even sometimes obligatory. This is an important distinction. It is a commonly held liberal view that if a person is making a self-regarding autonomous choice, it is always, all things considered, wrong to interfere paternalistically with this choice, irrespective of the benefits of the

---

[9] If a reason supports my decision to do something, then I have a '*pro-tanto*' reason to do it: it is '*pro tanto*' (i.e. to that extent) right for me to do it.

interference to the person's life. For instance, imagine that you have shared with me that you are struggling to decide what you want to do with your life: you want to train as a psychoanalyst, but your family think you should go into investment banking, and you are experiencing a lot of stress because of this. I could give you a tablet, unbeknownst to you, that would relieve you of the painful indecision and make you opt for a career in psychoanalysis because, in this hypothetical example, I know beyond doubt that you would have a better life than if you pursued a career in investment banking. On this view, this paternalistic action is nevertheless wrong because it interferes with your autonomous decision, even if my intervention would make your life go better. In other words, giving beneficence primacy over patient autonomy can amount to paternalism.

Yet, we will all recognize that some clinical situations cannot be dealt with simplistically by giving primacy to autonomy. We sometimes must ask ourselves if it is ethical to stop a patient making an unwise choice, one that will predictably cause him to suffer significant harm. In turn, these considerations beg the thorny question of what justifies the epistemic superiority of certain people to determine when others are 'mistaken' about their own interests and self-understanding. I touched on this issue in Chapter 1, and by now it will be clearer that we are faced with a difficult ethical challenge: how can a therapist be better placed to know than the patient? Do we have a right to deprive someone of their autonomy, for example, to enhance well-being over time as we define it?

In terms of the law, and intervention by the state, one oft-cited response to this dilemma draws on an important liberal principle articulated by John Stuart Mill. Mill's so-called 'harm principle' claims that the only justification for infringing the liberties of an individual is to prevent harm to others (i.e. an intervention in a person's other-regarding actions); harm to the self does not suffice (i.e. an intervention in a person's self-regarding actions). This belief underpins Mill's concept of 'temporary intervention': we can intervene to ascertain *whether* a person is acting autonomously. For example, as therapists we do sometimes restrict a person's liberty when we are involved in activating the process of being sectioned under the Mental Health

Act. There are no 'right' answers to these clinical dilemmas, yet part of our ethical responsibility is to engage with these questions in our mind and be prepared for the complexity of the decisions we may have to make, and that all too often we are called to make under pressure in response to a crisis.

One final consideration is due with respect to autonomy. The principle of respect for autonomy underpins the requirement for valid *consent to treatment*. Often what passes for patient autonomy in medical care settings is 'operationalised by practices of informed consent' (O'Neill, 2002: 38), which engage the patient in evaluating cost-benefit questions. I am of the view that in routine psychoanalytic practice (especially in the private sector) we do not give sufficient consideration with the patient to these questions when we offer to work with him. However, I am sympathetic to the challenge we face as therapists: consent should not be reduced to a form of consumer protectionism, which in medical settings insists, for example, on full disclosure of risks, preferably based on follow-up studies of how such risks have worked, or not, in past interventions. This approach is referred to as 'protectionist bioethics' and it takes for granted the presuppositions of consumerism; thus, it wants people to know exactly what is being delivered at what cost and with what risk. The ethical standards are liberal, turning medical professionals into 'responsible' salespeople and then leaving the choice to patient-consumers (Candilis et al., 2018).

One (of several) problem with this project is the difficulty of accurately specifying the potential benefits, costs, and risks, not least for a process as unique as psychoanalytic psychotherapy or psychoanalysis. Moreover, there are legitimate concerns, for example, about how much a very emotionally distressed patient can take in at the end of a psychotherapy assessment to enable meaningful consent. However, we should bear in mind that 'taking in' a diagnosis of cancer is also emotionally demanding and yet we would still expect the doctor to share the treatment options with their associated risks but anticipate that this may need to be revisited in the next appointment to ensure understanding. Similarly, consent to psychoanalytic therapy may not be most usefully conceptualized as a one-off event but rather as a process whereby the patient can only begin to gain a realistic sense of the nature of therapy through experiencing it. It's clear that we face important challenges to seeking consent that reflect the unique nature of the analytic encounter. However, such legitimate concerns do not obviate the need to provide patients with some information about the type of therapy we offer and the alternatives. The clinical challenge is *how* we create the conditions for consent with a new patient in a meaningful manner.

Justice

Matters of the 'good' concern ethics whereas matters of the 'right' concern justice. The norms of justice are thought to be universally binding, that is they hold independent of people's commitments to specific values. Justice is, simply put, giving to each his due. As a concept, it refers to fairness, equality, and equitable[10] treatment. If we work in a publicly funded service, where resource allocation is a more tangible reality that impacts on individual patients and on the therapist's capacity to deliver a service, justice considerations will be more than familiar.

Of the several categories of justice, the one that is most pertinent to clinical ethics is *distributive justice*. The principle of distributive justice requires being just and fair to all patients and respecting their human rights and dignity. Justice, as fair treatment to all, concerns the distribution of scarce health resources, and the decision of who gets what treatment. This involves determining impartially the provision of services for patients and the allocation of services between them. There are different valid principles of distributive justice such as on the basis of an equal share or according to need or to effort, to name but a few. Each principle is not exclusive, and can be, and is often, combined in application. It is easy to see the difficulty in

[10] *Equality* refers to how we should all be treated in the same manner, irrespective of any individual differences. *Equity* refers to how we should all be provided with what we need to succeed.

choosing, balancing, and refining these principles to form a coherent and workable solution to distribute psychotherapeutic resources, but this is not the focus here.

At first glance, considerations of distributive justice will seem far removed from the preoccupations of the private practice clinician. In psychotherapy, we are more oriented towards the treatment of the individual patient, rather than to thinking about resource distribution among the broader population. On closer inspection, however, the principle of justice is also relevant to private practice, but this is not always recognized. Because justice is generally interpreted as fair treatment of persons, this principle is therefore highly relevant to psychotherapy. Considerations of justice are centrally implicated when we evaluate any clinical decision because we must ask whether our actions treat all persons equally. If not, the onus is on us to determine whether the difference in treatment is justified. For example, is our respect for absolute confidentiality more nuanced when working with some patients? Are we more inclined to insist on writing to the General Practitioner (doctor) with some patients but waive this request more readily if the patient has a public profile and does not want any trace on his medical records of psychological problems? Or consider how we respond to patient requests outside of the session frame: are we implicitly biased to respond more promptly to the patient who is more articulate and/or insistent, who feels perhaps more entitled because they pay us a high fee? Or is our response determined by our assessment of the complexity of the case? Or do we explicitly operate on a policy of equal time for every patient or have a blanket policy that we do not respond out of session times? When we are referred a patient, whose clinical presentation is less familiar to us and we know of a colleague who is more experienced in this area, but we decide nevertheless to take the patient on, perhaps because we are curious to learn more about their presenting problem, is this fair to the patient? Consider too how when there is a lot of demand for our services, and we have the possibility of selecting who we take into our practice, on what basis do we make the selection? Is it based on the patients we find most interesting, the ones who can pay us more, the ones who are least emotionally demanding? Finally let's look at the example of uninsured patients: when we decide to *not* offer a vacancy to a non-insured patient who cannot afford the higher end private fee on our scale, and instead we offer the space to someone who is insured and thus covers a higher fee, we are making an ethical decision that we could argue is not 'just' in so far as we are treating the two patients differently based on the fee they can afford. I am not suggesting that there is a morally right answer to this kind of dilemma but merely that it is important that we recognize it as an ethical decision that concerns matters of justice.

This is but a small sample of the many challenging ethical questions that invite us to think about whether we treat all potential patients fairly and equally. In answering these questions, it is important to do so keeping in mind the difference between what we think we should ideally do and what we do in practice. In some instances, the discrepancy between the two can be large. Our decisions with respect to these matters reflect our values and our desires. We are more protected from the 'backstory' to these ethical decisions when we have more limited freedom around our work, for example when we work for an institution that pays us. However, when we can make more choices and/or accountability stops with us, considerations of justice come to the fore and are deeply challenging. Such questions invite us to keep in mind that as therapists we are responsible for preventing unjust practices through remaining aware of our biases and of the strengths and limits of our expertise. It is incumbent on us to clarify the basis for justifying differential treatment and whether our reasons hold. After all, it is relatively easy to identify reasons for why we act as we do but not all reasons are equal in their ethical merit or coherence.

Fairness to the patient assumes a primary importance when there are conflicts of interests. An example of a violation of the principle of justice is when a particular option of treatment, such as a long-term, open-ended, individual psychoanalytic therapy, is recommended over others, such as group analytic therapy, which may be equally effective and a less expensive option for the patient. If we recommend the long-term individual therapy option, it is essential to pause to consider if this is because we have good reasons to believe that of all the options, this is the one that benefits the patient most or whether it benefits us, perhaps because we have a vacancy we need to fill and we don't offer group therapy or because the patient is of particular interest to us and we want the experience. Perhaps we consider that they are both equally valid interventions, in which case we then need to ensure that we discuss the relative costs and benefits of each one with the patient to ensure valid consent.

A commitment to fairness also requires us to appreciate differences between people and to be committed to equality of opportunity, avoiding discrimination against people or groups. Every patient must get fair treatment irrespective of ethnic background, gender, sexuality, religion, or disability. Ensuring fair treatment rests on our capacity to attend to issues of power and authority experienced in the unconscious as part of the analytic process. This necessitates reflection on our own identity, culture, values, preconceptions, and worldview and the impact of these on the analytic relationship and process. Awareness and understanding of a patient's demographic characteristics are essential but we must also be mindful of the *intersectionality* of such factors. Intersectionality as a concept was introduced by the legal theorist Kimberlé Crenshaw (1991) as a way of understanding the multidimensional crossover points of oppression. Intersectionality is a sociological paradigm that suggests that oppression is not based solely on race, ethnicity, gender, class, religion, or socio-economic status but results from the interaction between these factors, which amounts to more than the sum of each of them. It has become a key concept for deconstructing forms of interpersonal power and authority. Its merit lies in the focus on multiple causal mechanisms resulting in an individual's oppression.[11]

For example, to return to the domestic abuse example cited earlier, the therapist working with a patient who discloses domestic abuse, in deliberating an ethical course of action, will need to understand the concept of intersectionality. The interaction of important demographic variables influences what resources are available

---

[11] For a critical discussion of how the concept may also be misused, see Pilgrim (2022).

to individuals, how accessible and/or affordable treatment will be, and how realistic it is to leave an abusive partner (Bograd, 1999). Intersectionality theory allows us to conceptualize how some low socio-economic-status minority women may feel that by reporting the abuse, they will be perpetuating a stereotype of their culture or that they may be at greater risk for losing custody of their children. Similarly, a therapist may not recognize the presence of violence if a woman does not fit into any of the categories that the therapist typically associates with violence. Such a bias would impact the fairness of the intervention with this particular patient.

This all too brief discussion of the relevance of intersectionality theory is in the service of a broader point: it is not simply that understanding such a theory is helpful or desirable but rather that it is an ethical requirement if we are to deliver an intervention that is fair to all. This is because it is essential to consider the unique factors that impact on a person's experience, such as in the previous example of domestic abuse, within specific socio-demographic groups. Traditionally psychoanalysis has privileged the focus on internal world dynamics, but external reality also must be factored in when we consider the ethics of our work. It is not a question of either/or but that both internal and external factors matter and interact in highly complex ways.

Impossible decisions: The use of specification and balancing

Clinical reality is far removed from the preceding outline of principles in abstract. Because we often have competing obligations, this poses a serious challenge in clinical contexts. Some moral theories regard it as incoherent that there could be contradictory obligations and argue that the only *ought* is the one generated by a higher order value (e.g. lying is *always* wrong). In this book, and in keeping with the approach adopted by Beauchamp and Childress (2013), I suggest that in clinical practice various moral principles, rules, and rights can and do conflict: such that 'What agents ought to do is . . . determined by what they ought to do *all things considered*' (Beauchamp and Childress, 2013: 15; my italics).

To reach an 'all things considered' position, the four principles need to be particularized enough to provide justification and guide action in the given clinical situation. Two crucial steps assist this process. The first is *specification*. This involves narrowing the scope of the principles involved and necessitates '... spelling out where, when, why, how, by what means, to whom, or by whom the action is to be done or avoided' (Beauchamp and Childress, 2013: 17). For example, we can specify the principle of justice by adopting a rule that prohibits only offering intensive psychotherapy based on the patient's cognitive abilities because learning difficulties need not be an obstacle though the way the therapist works may require adaptations. Specifications are required to guide actions: respect for autonomy, as we saw in the previous section, is too vague. Whether autonomy trumps other principles will depend on other factors, such as the patient's age or mental state.

The second important process is *balancing*. It often happens that multiple norms collide with one another and favour competing courses of action in a particular situation. In *The Right and the Good*, the Scottish moral philosopher, W. D. Ross (1930) distinguished between so-called *prima facie duties* and *actual duties*. A prima facie duty must be fulfilled unless in conflict with an equal or stronger duty. An *actual duty* requires examining the respective weights of competing prima facie duties. According to Ross, a prima facie duty is a duty that is binding or obligatory, other things being equal. Common examples include the duty to tell the truth, obey the law, protect people from harm, and keep one's promises. For therapists this would mean, for example, that we should not lie to patients about the circumstances in their lives or falsify records about them. These are duties we ought to perform, in and of themselves, other things being equal.

Sometimes it is clear which competing prima facie principle is stronger, but there are many situations where it is very difficult to tell which principle is the most stringent, all-things-considered obligation. For example, if in the therapist's opinion a very suicidal patient requires hospital admission but the patient refuses to go voluntarily, the therapist must judge whether beneficence or respect for autonomy is the weightier norm. Even a rule such as 'put the patient's interests first', is not absolute when we consider possible conflicts with other commitments in a variety of circumstances. Balancing is the attempt to determine the comparative weight and priority of moral principles in particular cases where they come into conflict, to reach a conclusion about which principle is the overriding consideration that ought to be followed.

A frequent challenge in psychotherapeutic practice is that 'other things' often are not equal. Moral philosophers refer to this as the *ceteris paribus*[12] problem. Often, we are confronted with scenarios where we should discharge one obligation and override another. Conflicts among prima facie duties constitute ethical dilemmas, that is, conflicts among one's moral duties and obligations. In psychotherapy we can be faced with a conflict between the prima facie duty to protect patient confidentiality and the prima facie duty to protect people, including patients and third parties, from harm. Breaches of confidentiality might be justified where we consider that the prevention of harm to the patient or a third party trumps the commitment to confidentiality. In assessing which risks to third parties outweigh rules or rights to confidentiality, the probability that the harm will materialize, and the magnitude of that harm must be balanced against the norms of confidentiality and the possible harms that might occur by breaching these norms.

Underlying tensions can emerge when faced with the dual imperatives of 'do good' and 'do no harm'. I want to illustrate this with an example taken from the expanding field of computer-mediated psychological interventions because it gives a sense of this ethical complexity. I also share the following example to underline the point that any ethical system that functions in a rote manner—whether it is mediated by a machine or an actual therapist—potentially exposes the patient to harm. Nowadays some online therapeutic sites

---

[12] This means 'all things being equal'.

deploy algorithms to manage the automated detection of 'at risk patients' who use these sites—this is an instance of the algorithm in the service—in theory—of 'doing good'. Psychoanalytically speaking we would argue that the opportunity for a patient to disclose and make sense of his suicidal thoughts can be very helpful (beneficence) and does not necessarily require action to be taken, such as involving psychiatric care, which might expose the patient to harm (maleficence). However, an algorithm cannot reliably differentiate adequately between a disclosure of suicidal thoughts that is therapeutic in nature, that is having disclosed this impulse the person feels relieved and is less likely to act on it, from one indicative of heightened risk requiring action. Such an algorithm would most likely be accompanied by a high rate of false positives resulting in inappropriate clinical intervention arising from an inaccurate interpretation of the individual's online behaviour. This could cause unintended harm by failing to respect a patient's perceived boundaries of privacy and autonomy.

The challenge therefore is how we make differential judgements rather than abide by uniform policies. Applying general rules to all patients may lead us to ignore the morally and clinically relevant features of different situations. When faced with the need to balance, we are also immediately confronted with the question of how much our intuitions can guide us through this process, or whether we need principles as a guide. An influential compromise was suggested by the political philosopher John Rawls (1973). He proposed that we should compare and combine our intuitive responses with theory and argument in a process called *reflective equilibrium*, which sets out the importance of bringing together principles, judgements, and background theories into a state of equilibrium or harmony. Rawls' idea is to look at where our intuitions and theory come together, and where they differ. When they pull in different directions, he suggests that we should re-examine both our intuitions (perhaps they are biased or represent a misunderstanding) and our theory (perhaps the theory is mistaken). This back-and-forth process might lead us to revise our initial feelings about a problem, as well as to revise our arguments and morals.

Beauchamp and Childress (2013) offer one solution to the balancing problem. First, they affirm that balancing is not just a matter of mere intuition or feeling, but of finding *good reasons* to justify specific judgments about the relative weight of conflicting principles. As I touched on earlier, this requires balancing and adjudicating between two 'goods'. Since we are not united by a shared view of the 'good', we will specify and balance the principles differently, hence the principlists' claim 'that there can be different and equally good solutions to moral problems' (Gordon et al., 2011: 299). For example, what do we do with a life support system for a patient in a permanent coma? Both removing it, and continuing it, are justified from different standpoints, and so appear equally good depending on whether we take an absolutist stance which gives more weight to the primacy of life or a utilitarian stance that favours giving a dignified exit to a life deemed no longer worth living.

In practice, ethical judgments boil down to decisions about which prima facie duties take priority or precedence when they conflict. While we might yearn for formulaic algorithms that tell us what to do when this is the case, the hard reality is that very often reasonable minds can and do differ about the 'right' course of action. The Four Principles approach does not purport to provide a method for dealing with irresoluble dilemmatic conflict of the principles or of the many more specific moral obligations encompassed by them. It merely systematizes how we might think about such dilemmas giving us a framework for considering the difference between prima facie and actual duties.

Balancing competing obligations requires us to consider what we ought to do and what we ought not to do, but we also need to consider what is *supererogatory*, that is those actions that go 'beyond the call of duty'. Broadly speaking, supererogatory acts are morally good although not (strictly) required. Professional roles engender obligations that do not bind persons who do not occupy these roles. For example, a therapist who suspects a child is being abused based on her assessment of a child in therapy with her, has a greater responsibility to act on this suspicion than the child's next-door neighbour who speculates about this same possibility based on her observations as a neighbour. This is not to suggest that the neighbour has no responsibility, only that the therapist's failure to act on her suspicions represents a clearer ethical failing given the responsibilities inherent to her training in these matters and the obligations inherent to her professional role in relation to the child.

However, we sometimes need to draw the line between what is ethically required given our role and what is supererogatory. Take the example of a therapist working with a very suicidal patient who has recently tried to kill himself. She is asked by the patient if he can reach out to her during her holiday break if he feels suicidal again. The patient is well known to the therapist and has experienced significant abuse in his life such that he finds it hard to trust easily. The therapist has put in place a 'crisis plan' for the patient to cover the break. So, the patient has access to help but not the specific help he prefers and that, we could argue, might be more effective given that the patient feels understood and contained by his therapist. This could be reasonably expected to be more desirable, possibly even more effective, than seeing someone who has never met the patient before or barely knows him.

In such a scenario, and from a transferential point of view, we might wonder about the meaning of the patient's request and what is being enacted if the therapist agreed to be available during her break. From an ethical point of view, we could argue convincingly that the therapist has more than discharged her obligations to the patient by identifying alternative support during her absence and she is entitled to a break—we might even argue that part of her ethical practice is to ensure that she does take breaks so that she protects her mental well-being and is better placed, overall, to help all her patients equally. However, this patient might not have the personal and/or interpersonal resources to avail himself of help from another person during the therapist's absence and his risk might well be enhanced during the break. Even so, under these circumstances, if the therapist decided to provide a crisis service to her patient, and irrespective of the countertransferential meaning of this decision, from an ethical point of view her actions during the break would most likely be understood to be supererogatory. To understand it as such does not relieve us of the emotional implications of the choice we make; it simply clarifies that we have made a choice based on some identifiable principles. Neither would the choice to see the patient during a break imply in any clear-cut sense that the therapist is any more virtuous than the therapist who would opt not to do this.

Principles over character?

By now it will be clear that life is far more complex than a principled approach can fully accommodate. Clinical reality does not allow for a formulaic approach. Any framework that elaborates general principles is likely to be unyielding to the demands of the specifics of the individual patient. For every ethical dilemma we face, or for every therapeutic intervention that we make, a range of important factors must be taken into consideration on a case-by-case basis. Even so, as the philosopher Onora O'Neill, observes:

> . . . it is true that we cannot expect any practical principles, whether legal or ethical, social technical, to provide a life algorithm. But the fact that principles underdetermine action means only that they must be complimented and implemented by the exercise of judgement, and practical input involving ethical judgement is not a matter of arbitrary choice. (O'Neill, 2002: 120)

Ethical judgement, as we have seen in this chapter, rests on the exercise of reflective equilibrium. This is the state we aim to cultivate as part of the *ethical chóros*, which helps us to consider the tensions between competing obligations. The state of reflective equilibrium could be redescribed psychoanalytically as a state of questioning our countertransference (used here in the narrow sense of the term), alert to the pressures potentially arising from allegiance to our 'idols of the cave' (see 'Introduction'), to our personal equation, and to our personal investments in certain values and norms, all of which might pull us away from serving the best interests of the patient. The state of back-and-forth questioning and revision is essential to the *ethical chóros* and to being able to identify guiding principles for our clinical decisions. This requires us to be clear about our duties. When we have a duty to do something, this means that we ought to do it, because it is our responsibility. The French philosopher Simone Weil (1952) took the strong view that duties are prior to rights. According to her, the effective exercise of the right springs not from the individual who possesses it but from other people who consider themselves as being under a certain obligation towards him. This forces us to consider the capabilities that agents and institutions need if they are to discharge their obligations and thereby respect one another's rights. Obligation shifts the focus from an individualistic way of thinking to one that takes the *relationship* between 'obligation bearers' and 'rights holders' to be central (O'Neill, 2002), a position that strikes a more congruent psychoanalytic chord and roots us back into the importance of the psychoanalytic promise.

In this chapter I have not addressed a virtue approach,[13] that is an approach to ethics that underscores the importance of character. Virtues are morally desirable dispositions of character. The centrality of character in professional ethics has received a lot of attention and reflects wider developments in contemporary ethics and moral philosophy that draw on Aristotle's ideas. These positions take issue with the view that moral deliberation and the justification for our decisions can proceed deductively through the application of general principles, as I have been describing so far. By contrast, Aristotle argued that the phenomena that concern ethical inquiry are mutable, indeterminate, and specific. As such, he believed that we cannot look to general principles of right action to settle what is the right thing to do. Instead, we must look to the character or virtues. This view was core to his discussion of *prudential wisdom*. Aristotle claimed that unlike scientific wisdom, which contemplates fixed truths, prudential wisdom requires grappling with phenomena that are variable and that require the careful study of particulars. This led him to stress the importance of *phronesis* (practical judgment), a practical reasoning skill that is neither a matter of simply applying general

[13] See Glossary for definition.

principles to particular cases nor of mere intuition. The *phronimos* is an expert practical reasoner.

Brenner and Cather (2015) argue for the relevance of such an approach to psychoanalytic practice rather than the elaboration of rules of conduct or moral principles. They emphasize the 'psychodynamic virtues' such as empathy and neutrality. I have no doubt that there is considerable merit in discussing 'communicative or relational virtues', as I would label them, such as patience, empathy, reciprocity, and tolerance. These are clearly fundamental to our work, but I am not persuaded that we can establish an adequate professional ethic based on the character of practitioners alone even though the latter is self-evidently very important. In isolation, the character approach cannot provide a sufficient grounding for the ethical obligations of therapists and, as I have also suggested, a principled approach cannot encompass the particularity of each case. Therefore, both are required. As Gillon proposes: 'Virtues . . . are needed both for moral obligations to be instantiated and sustained in the moral life of real people and for all sorts of other supererogatory but morally desirable aspects of life' (2003: 309). Consideration of both general principles and of the idiosyncratic features of the experiences presented by a patient play a role in phronesis such that the therapist's judgment *and* character are clearly central to the process.

Ethical principles emerge from commonalities embodied in concrete human circumstances. Indeed, Aristotle identified the ability to recognize and be guided by such principles as an essential capacity of the prudent person. Without this we would be lost in a sea of unrelated particulars with no ability to anticipate or plan an ethically sound course for the ethical decisions we face in the consulting room. Exercising the *ethical chóros* relies on our attuned and skilled responsiveness to both the patient's shifting internal and external contexts, as much as our own, drawing on the core ethical principles outlined in this chapter as touchpoints in our thinking about what is best for the patient, keeping in mind the contextual nature of ethical dilemmas. This requires that we consider how the bioethical principles we have reviewed so far can be integrated within a specifically psychoanalytic framework, which is the focus of Chapter 3.

3

A Psychoanalytic Principled Approach

Thou canst not touch the freedom of my mind.
—(John Milton, 1634)

In Chapter 2 I outlined the Four Principles model drawn from bioethics. I suggested that it provides a systematic framework for helping us to question the ethics of our interventions and for thinking through the plethora of clinical dilemmas that we encounter in our consulting rooms. Not only can psychoanalytic work benefit from this framework but also psychoanalysis allows us to add specificity and complexity to the principles due to its appreciation of unconscious mentation and relational dynamics. In this chapter, I delineate a conceptual structure that can accommodate bioethical principles compatible with a model of the mind that subscribes to unconscious mentation, and I contextualize this for use in everyday psychoanalytic practice. In addition to the Four Principles, I propose the addition of a fifth one—veracity—that is central to psychoanalytic work.

Before I set out to meet my aims for this chapter, I must name the proverbial elephant: it is impossible to discuss the ethics of psychoanalytic practice without specifying what it is that we do. The challenge of this task will be obvious. How can we even begin to consider what would constitute specifically psychoanalytic beneficent or maleficent actions without a working model of the purpose of the analytic encounter and what the therapist strives to offer, at her best? The different schools of psychoanalysis place different emphases on the aims of psychotherapy or psychoanalysis, with some therapists probably rejecting the very notion of an 'aim' as appropriate to the analytic endeavour. Even where there is agreement over the question of aims, the different traditions hold notoriously divergent views about how to best facilitate these aims (e.g. through the interpretation of the transference or the analysis of defence). It is well beyond the scope of this book to engage in these debates. However, to the extent that there are many versions of what psychoanalysis is and what it is not, this poses a considerable challenge to my attempt to reinterpret the ethical principles in a psychoanalytic frame.

I cannot meaningfully discuss ethical principles without a unifying starting point about what we are aiming to do as psychoanalytic practitioners. In this respect I am indebted to Dominique Scarfone's (2017) inspiring call to ethics as a way of distilling the essence of our work and so bypassing the in-house politics of divergent views about the nature of psychoanalysis. Finding some common ground across psychoanalytic schools of thought through consideration of the 'ethics of translation', as he puts it, resonates with the challenge I face in this chapter. However, since this old psychoanalytic chestnut is not the primary driver for this book, I have taken the easier path, in one sense, and will present my own elaboration of what I think I aim to do with my patients and articulate what I perceive to be the common ground uniting psychoanalytic practice. This rightly opens me to criticism: it is an idiosyncratic take on psychoanalysis and ethics, and I don't expect agreement.[1] Yet, I hope that it can at least act as a catalyst for a discussion of how we might introduce ethics more systematically into our trainings. No matter what you make of my personal stance, the take-home message is nevertheless generalizable: consideration of the nature and aspirations of psychoanalytic interventions is part of the ethical work. This is the starting point of any discussion about its ethics, and hence it is also what we should prioritize reflecting upon in our trainings. This chapter is an

---

[1] This is a personal view, but it is nevertheless informed by the systematic review that I led on the development of psychoanalytic competences (Lemma et al., 2008). To this extent, it is rooted in some assumptions that met with the expert consensus and with research evidence.

illustration of this process with my position used as an example. It is not intended to be an assertion that '*this* is psychoanalysis'.

The telos of psychoanalytic work

The value-laden nature of psychoanalysis

Aristotle believed that everything has a purpose or 'final end'. This is what he referred to as the *telos*. In ethical theory, each human action is taken to be directed towards a *telos*. Whether the aim is explicit or not, at the outset patient and therapist agree to meet to help the patient with 'something', even if this 'something' may be loosely defined as 'expanding self-understanding', for example (Blass, 2003). The patient will understand that the therapy session has some purpose even if it may not yet be ripe for verbal articulation. The therapist will also have her own position on what it is that she is hoping to do for and with the patient even though many therapists never discuss this openly with the patient at the assessment stage or beyond— something that, as we saw in Chapter 2, raises important ethical questions around consent to engaging in an analytic process.

Some psychoanalytic practitioners prefer to eschew the thorny question of 'cure' and/or argue that 'cure' is not what psychoanalysis aims for.[2] We are still debating whether psychoanalysis is a form of 'treatment' (Puget, 2017). It is valid to argue that a cure-based model of the psychoanalytic endeavour is inadequate, but this position does not discharge us from the requirement to specify our aims or why it is not appropriate to work towards a *telos*: it merely clarifies that for some therapists, 'cure' is not the aim. The aims of the therapist are often implicit. This is ethically compromising. I suggest that we are on dangerous ground when we believe that the direction of a psychoanalytic process is not informed by (often implicit) notions

---

[2] See, for example, Robert Caper's (1999) interesting discussion of this: '. . . only by resisting the urge to achieve a cure with an interpretation can the analyst discharge his primary responsibility to the patient, which is not to heal him, but to help him recover himself' (1999: 26).

of what is and is not healthy or of what constitutes 'mature development'.[3] These notions are embedded in psychoanalytic developmental theory, which inevitably informs what we take up and focus on with the patient even if we don't explicitly acknowledge this. We face a complex challenge because we enter the analytic encounter with considerable 'baggage'. We all have values that guide how we approach our work given our own developmental experiences, education, cultural, and socio-economic background. Our role requires us to bracket these so that we can attend to the patient's individuality. We also work with a model of the mind that, no matter which way we square it, is steeply embedded in *normative* ideals. The very notion of 'psychopathology' that lies at the core of psychoanalytic developmental models is an ethical concept because it raises value questions.

The philosopher Edward Harcourt draws attention to the implicit normative contrast in descriptions about the paranoid-schizoid and depressive positions, noting how '. . . the move from the paranoid-schizoid to the depressive position is envisaged not only as a normal maturational step, but as a moral improvement' (2018: 129). I enthusiastically encourage you to read this paper where you will find his arguments to support this position, which I evidently share. For our purposes, I want to simply emphasize that we are all influenced by theories of the mind that frame some ways of being in the world as more desirable than others. If we work with a patient who shows little or no concern for other people, and whom we might say functions in a predominantly paranoid-schizoid fashion, I imagine that in addition to trying to understand why he may need to operate in this manner, and striving not to be judgemental, most therapists will focus their interventions in the direction of supporting more depressive position functioning (assuming this is the model of the mind they subscribe to). Similarly, if we observe a patient humiliating

---

[3] I concur with Barratt (2015) when he argues that ethics and morality are not the same, but this is where my agreement with his position ends. He proposes that psychoanalysis distinguishes itself by establishing a healing relationship that is both ethical and amoral and strongly cautions against directing a patient 'towards an ideal of mature and adaptive functioning' (2012: 1). Although he is right that it is not our role to 'direct' our patients, we must recognize the normative assumptions embedded in our psychoanalytic theories and which inevitably shape our interventions.

those close to him, including us in the transference, when in the grip of a pathological superego, the focus of our interventions will most likely be informed by a belief that it is best for the patient to establish contact with '. . . an object with *normal* superego aspects' (O'Shaughnessy, 1999: 869; my italics) that supports '. . . the operation of *normal* ethics' (O'Shaughnessy, 1999: 869; my italics). Or when we aim more broadly to support mentalizing in the patient, we are asserting its value and desirability, perhaps because we believe that mentalizing encourages reciprocity in relationships (Allen, 2008), and these are 'goods' that we value. In other words, whichever psychoanalytic theory we subscribe to, it is steeped in assumptions about health, pathology, and the 'good' life. As such we cannot sidestep the reality that we work to an overarching aim—the broad direction we believe healthy development needs to take—even if we do not explicitly articulate this much of the time:

> Psychoanalysis can hardly fail to be interested in the difference between a life's going well and its going not so well, so—though some analysts are, for historical reasons, still allergic to the mere word—it must involve some 'ethics of the good'. (Harcourt, 2018: 146)

What we selectively focus on in our interventions implicitly steers the patient towards ways of being consistent with the perceived to be more 'healthy' or 'adaptive' states of mind.[4] To the extent that this is true, then we are discussing matters of morality. Whilst some clinicians might disagree with this, others such as Meissner describe very clearly the sleight of mind when we claim that psychoanalysis is not a moral enterprise:

> If I diagnose a patient as having paranoid tendencies, have I also made a judgment regarding the moral or ethical status of the patient? At a

---

[4] Alert to the risk that this poses, Freud was wise to remind us that,

> . . . however much the analyst may be tempted to become a teacher, model and ideal for other people and create men in his own image, he should not forget that . . . he will be disloyal to his task if he allows himself to be led on by such inclinations . . . . In all his attempts at improving and educating the patient the analyst should respect his individuality. (1938: 175)

minimum, I am making a judgment about the quality of the patient's psychic organization and about the defensive pattern of his reactions to his personal and social environment. There is something wrong, faulty, maladaptive about the way in which the patient's personality is organized and functions. There is implicit a value judgment that to be some other way is better and more acceptable than the way the patient is. The analyst in such a case is implicitly positing a standard or ideal of personality integration and functioning that he holds as normative in the process of establishing his diagnosis. (Meissner, 1994: 456)

There is an important difference between being nonjudgemental or neutral in our response to what a patient reports and who he aspires to become and claiming that we are neutral when it comes to what we believe makes a life go well. The former is an ethically sound aspiration; the latter is, in my view, an impossibility. Let me put it more strongly: claiming to be value-free and disavowing our investments in specific and valued ways of being in the world is a dangerous myth insofar as it makes the value judgments upon which therapy is based inaccessible to conscious evaluation and eventual bracketing and, as such, can work to undermine the patient's autonomy. We are wise to question ourselves if we perceive a leaning towards becoming 'moral entrepreneurs' (Barratt, 2015: 2) and so corrupting the analytic stance. But we must not ignore our biases and values as they invariably impact on our practice. Bion's call to approach each session 'without memory or desire' is an important reminder that we need to remain vigilant to the inevitable intrusions of our needs, desires, and psychoanalytic agendas, not that we can eliminate them in any absolute sense.

Analytic listening is demanding precisely because it requires that we listen without regard to the filter of fixed identities or succumbing to the allure of seemingly neutral and reasonable normalizing discourses that assign to the patient a nature that is exempt from contingency and outside history. When the cornerstones of our seemingly stable but in fact provisional identities or our expectations of what is 'normal' loosen or crumble, we may reach out for the comforts of psychoanalytic theories that provide a familiar orientation. In so doing we may fail to recognize the many aspects of life in which we each have vested interests, and how these create potential obstacles to how we listen and respond to our patients (Kirshner, 2012).

Developing a mind of one's own

I took a detour into the question of values because inevitably the articulation of the *telos* of psychoanalytic work that I will propose shortly reflects my personal analytic journey, preferences, and values. That said, having undergone three analyses and supervisions with analysts from three different schools of psychoanalysis (Freudian, Kleinian, and Independent), and through my involvement in the work on articulating the competences for the practice of psychoanalytic psychotherapy (Lemma et al., 2008), I have been fortunate to sample differences and overlaps across several analytic traditions. I take these privileged (and very helpful) experiences as a viewing point from which to propose an overarching *telos* that does not make too many demands on core metapsychological assumptions, namely that the 'final end' of psychoanalytic work (Lear, 2009) is to facilitate the patient's development of a mind of his own, to help him to better understand what he is and what he is not, to evaluate the functions and costs of his defensive structures on himself and on his relationships, thereby supporting relational autonomy. When we have a sense of our own mind, of its blind spots and characteristic defences, of its unique ways of shoring up self-esteem and managing strong affects, of our conscious and unconscious desires, needs, hopes, and anxieties, we can begin to change how we exist with others in ways that make our lives go better. Clearly, the quality of our relationships, hence how we treat others, is central to my vision of what makes a life go better.[5]

---

[5] At the heart of the individual psyche is the imprint of the other. Intersubjective life is the context in which we develop, and we fall. The otherness that resides within the self requires understanding and management. Developing a mind of one's own is therefore central to the quality of our relationships. Without wishing to be reductionistic, what typically triggers the search for psychotherapy is manifest in, and often is consequent to or modulated by, what happens in our interpersonal worlds. This has been my repeated clinical experience even if the

Thomas Ogden's (2019) distinction between what he calls Freudian and Kleinian *epistemological psychoanalysis* (focused on knowing and understanding) and Winnicottian and Bionian *ontological psychoanalysis* (focused on being and becoming) underpins my position which, as will no doubt be clear to you by now, views the aim of the analytic process as that of helping the patient 'to become more fully himself' (Ogden, 2019: 664) through helping him to construct and know his mind, that is by strengthening the patient's representational (i.e. mentalizing) capacities, not only by motivating insight, though the latter is also important.[6] Where we place more or less emphasis through our interventions will depend on the patient and/or phase of a treatment.

The analytic process, as I understand it, aims to help the patient to develop a mind of his own through loosening (a) the grip of the developmental moorings which account for his (overdetermined) relational and affective patterns and (b) the grip of the knowledge he has of himself when he begins an analytic journey, which may be limiting or restricting in various ways. Through the analytic relationship, and its focus on assisting the development of his mind, the patient's unique relational, affective, and epistemic coordinates are articulated (i.e. made explicit) and reconfigured. I frame the aims in these terms specifically to highlight that the analytic encounter is one in which, when things go well, the patient acquires *epistemic goods* that support the development of autonomy. It is important ethically to recognize this, and I will return to this point when we consider the principle of psychoanalytic non-maleficence. In foregrounding epistemic goods, I am not suggesting that we are facilitating a cognitive

---

so-called problem presents at first as 'depression' or 'anxiety'. This is my starting presumption about why people most commonly seek therapy. From this derives what I believe we are aiming to do when we help people psychoanalytically, that is we are helping them to understand their own mind so that they can use this understanding to exist with others in ways that enhance individual, and ideally also collective, well-being.

[6] Ogden is clear that it is important

to bear in mind . . . that *there is no such thing as ontological psychoanalysis or epistemological psychoanalysis in pure form*. They coexist in mutually enriching relationship with one another. They are ways of thinking and being—sensibilities, not 'schools' of analytic thought or sets of analytic principles or analytic techniques. (2019: 662; italics in original)

process: epistemic goods are, in one sense, fundamentally relational goods in so far as we acquire them through dialogue with others. Moreover, some of these 'goods' refer to implicit relational experiences within the analytic encounter that can be transformative because they change our relational knowledge, that is what we have come to know and believe about ourselves and others.

If the *telos* is to support the development of 'a mind of one's own',[7] in the sense I outlined previously, and we can broadly agree on this descriptively, it's a start but not sufficient for our present purposes. We are concerned here with *psychoanalytic* work and hence with a model of the mind that recognizes the significance in mental life of an unconscious mind. So, we must also agree that developing a mind of one's own requires addressing nonconscious aspects of mental life. This presumption is not at all controversial in our discipline but suffice to say that it cannot reveal the techniques that are best suited to this end. My argument does not require their specification. I want to focus instead on two psychoanalytic assumptions that, I suggest, can cut across theoretical divides and are relevant to the ethics of our work because they concern the core of the psychoanalytic method. They are both obvious and uncontroversial, but it is important to set them out as a reminder of foundational points of potential convergence. Both these assumptions emerged clearly through the systematic evaluation of the competences required for the practice of psychoanalytic therapy. This work was based on the study of manualized therapies and cross-referenced with both the originators of various psychoanalytic models and with a psychoanalytic 'expert reference group' comprising representatives of different psychoanalytic traditions (Lemma et al., 2008). Consensus was reached on two features considered distinctive of a psychoanalytic approach, namely (a) the importance of the use of the relationship between patient and therapist to facilitate the work and (b) the importance of attending to unconscious processes. I therefore draw on these two assumptions as

---

[7] Although this expression is widely used, it was Robert Caper's (1999) text by this same title that consolidated it in my own mind.

unifying meta premises. Let me briefly expand on both in the service of clarity.

First, as psychoanalytic practitioners we most likely can agree that the primary vehicle for our work is the relationship between therapist and patient—one that is both bounded because it is a professional relationship yet limitless in the scope that it can give the patient for the elaboration of his mind. It is this that has important implications for psychoanalytic ethics: *we*—as individual subjects with our unique 'personal equation' (see Chapter 1), for better and for worse—mediate this work through the way we manage our own mind, and, in turn, this allows the patient to make 'use' of us. This does not make any presumptions about *how* the relationship is useful but merely *that* it is fundamental to the work.[8] Indeed, to what extent this unique relationship is used, and how it is used, varies as is apparent in different iterations of 'working in the transference'.[9]

Second, we can agree that the analytic relationship operates on both conscious and unconscious levels and therefore our work requires us to attend to both levels of experience within this relationship. Effectively, and to put it very simply, I am underlining that there are two people in a room, where one has the explicit role to help the other to understand his mind, and that this 'help' is inevitably mediated—first and foremost—by the person of the therapist, irrespective of the specific techniques she deploys to 'make use' of this relationship (e.g. transference interpretation, extra-transference interpretation, or a supportive intervention informed by a formulation of the transference). I am further specifying that this 'making use of' the relationship is psychoanalytic *only* if it includes consideration of the operation of an unconscious mind. It is vital to specify the latter given that many other types of psychotherapy also privilege the therapeutic relationship but don't attend to dynamically

---

[8] For example, in the work on competences, a clear distinction was also drawn between 'using the transference' as a constant backdrop in our minds that helps us to track who we have become in the patient's experience at a given juncture and 'interpreting the transference' as an active technique.

[9] Where we encounter more agreement, I think, is also with respect to the importance of protecting from external impingements what Jérome Glas has aptly termed the therapist's 'ethical status as object of the patient's psychic reality' (2021: 482).

or procedurally unconscious aspects of the unfolding therapeutic process—an example of this would be Interpersonal Psychotherapy (Lemma et al., 2009).

The two assumptions I have set out transcend the variegated ways in which psychoanalytic clinicians understand the analytic relationship and how it facilitates change. They do not rest on the assumption that it is primarily, as Scarfone suggests, 'the handling of transference [that] is a major and possibly a uniquely distinctive feature of our trade' (2017: 396). This is an important distinction between my position and that outlined by Scarfone even though he is qualified and measured in his own discussion about the transference. Even so, I am not specifying the 'handling of the transference' as the distinguishing feature of our work because of all the theoretical and technical baggage that flows from that claim. For my restricted purposes here, I am merely specifying that we work through the relationship that evolves between therapist and patient, that we acknowledge conscious and unconscious aspects to this relationship, including the operation of the transference relationship but not only, and that therapist's unique personal equation impacts on the evolution of this relationship.

A psychoanalytically informed principled framework

The specificity of our method, namely that we work through the relationship that develops between therapist and patient, means that the person of the therapist is thus central to its integrity and outcome. Recognizing this is fundamental to ethical practice because from this fact derive our ethical obligations towards the patient. In other words, what is relevant to our consideration of psychoanalytic ethics is that if (a) our overreaching telos is to help the patient to develop a mind of his own, and (b) our method requires the active use of the therapist's self to facilitate the patient's use of the therapist (in the service of the elaboration of a mind of his own), then (c) the ethical principles are in the service of protecting the conditions under which this work can be carried out for the benefit of the patient and without obstructing the process and/or harming the patient.

As I suggested in Chapter 1, we will all, at some point fall short of our aspiration to limit the bad and to maximally benefit the patient. This is so irrespective of how long our training analysis was or with whom or how experienced we are. To suggest that the therapist can somehow achieve a privileged position in relation to her own unconscious is 'an ethical sleight of hand' (Kirshner, 2012: 1231). Rather, the very nature of psychoanalytic work, because its method relies on the use of the therapist's self within the boundaries of the analytic setting, implies that thinking about ethics must squarely focus on the person of the therapist. I suggest that this highlights that one of our core responsibilities is our constant monitoring of countertransference, used in the restricted sense that I outlined in Chapter 1,[10] namely our desires, conflicts, and anxieties—our blind spots. In other words, the biggest risk in our work, and thus to the patient, is our 'opacity' to ourselves (Butler, 2005) and the shared tendency towards self-deception.

The self-monitoring[11] that I am advocating is an ethical labour, which is distinct from the contemporary use of countertransference as part of technique. A return to the use of countertransference in the original Freudian sense foregrounds that ethical practice requires the therapist's ongoing commitment to managing her own mind and to examining how through this she can support, inhibit, or damage the opportunities for the patient to discover his own mind and function autonomously. An implication of this for a psychoanalytic ethic is that the therapist has a *duty of self-knowledge*. Kant claimed that we are all under obligation to know ourselves. For Kant, the obligation to 'know myself' is a matter of knowing my moral character and progress towards the good (Ware, 2009). To put this in terms relevant to psychoanalytic practice, the obligation is to know our character[12] and how our personal equation promotes or inhibits

---

[10] See also Wilson (2020) for his excellent exposition of these ideas.

[11] This subsumes both self-reflexivity and self-reflection (see Chapter 1.

[12] I use the term character here in the broader sense of knowing about our characterological dispositions and associated defences but clearly this includes our moral character.

the patient's progress towards what he values and believes will make his life go better. My duty is to recognize what belongs to me—in so far as I can—so that I face squarely whether, for example, in making an interpretation, I have placed the pursuit of my values and narcissism above the pursuit of the patient's therapeutic ends. Questions like this force me to consider my unique position not only as a therapeutic agent but also as a moral agent. Being a moral agent does not need to mean that we are here to guide our patients morally, but that at the very least we have a requirement to know ourselves so that we can evaluate the all too often implicit value-led nature of our actions, which might include steering the patient in the direction of what we consider to be healthy but may not be of value to the patient. This is a central consideration for the psychoanalytic endeavour because we are responsible for not impinging upon the patient's development of an autonomous mind.

If I highlight the importance of monitoring the therapist's blind spots and the personal equation, I do not wish thereby to suggest that this requires a technical approach in which the therapist routinely discloses to the patient her countertransference. Although I am not concerned in this book with questions of technique, but with ethical ones, the two are inextricable from one another.[13] Suffice it to say that the issue at stake here is the importance of marking when something has gone wrong in the analytic relationship, the willingness to approach this non-defensively, and to take responsibility—themes that will be elaborated further in Chapter 6 when we discuss the 'Duty of Candour'. For now, it's enough to clarify that this is not the same as advocating self-disclosure as a technique.

---

[13] We cannot separate out discussions about technique (i.e. how we support the patient's therapeutic aims) from ethics. Scarfone notes the inseparable nature of technique and ethics:

'The analyst's know-how about conducting a psychoanalytic session is inseparable from his availability, which gives him the capacity to attend to a dimension of what occurs that is specific to psychoanalysis. How is this availability attained? Freud thought of it in technical terms when he spoke of evenly suspended attention, but I suggest it implies something more deeply seated in the analyst's attitude than a simple procedure. It requires of the analyst to accept being subjected to an experience without judging or trying to master what will happen—a kind of 'purposeful passivity', which in turn implies letting the patient guide the analyst all the while the analyst takes the responsibility of keeping the frame in place and the process going (2017: 395–396).

Let's now turn specifically to a psychoanalytic formulation of the bioethical principles I introduced in Chapter 2. I schematically set this out in Figure 3.1. This is intended to show how the Four Principles translate psychoanalytically with specifications that, I am suggesting, are core to the practice of psychoanalytic therapy. The model as summarized in Figure 3.1 will only make sense once the whole chapter has been read. It is intended as a summary of the whole chapter.

Relational autonomy

I place respect for the patient's *autonomy* as a central ethical consideration and at the heart of the proposed psychoanalytic ethics model. I echo the medical ethicist, Raanan Gillon's view that autonomy is the 'first amongst equals' (Gillon, 2003: 307) in terms of the ethical principles that should guide our interventions. I emphasize the respect for autonomy because the ability to think, to discriminate our conscious and unconscious wishes, desires, and anxieties, and make decisions about the way we want to lead our life based on self-understanding, and then to act on those decisions, is not only essential for mental health; it is also what makes ethical conduct possible, as Gillon suggests. For him, this is reason alone to state that autonomy therefore 'ought not merely to be respected, but its development encouraged and nurtured' (2003: 311). To the extent that I believe this to be true, it will be clear, as I outlined earlier, that I take it for granted that our values are inextricably woven into the analytic relationship.[14]

In discussing the importance of respecting and supporting the patient's autonomy, I mean specifically *relational* autonomy. I want

---

[14] I am touching only obliquely on the important question of whether therapy is at core about ethical development, but others have written eloquently about this, and I will not develop this theme further (see, for example, Drozek, 2019). However, even if, for the sake of argument, we do not believe that a core aim of therapy is to support the patient's ethical development, this does not therefore mean that our values do not impact the course of an analytic process.

THE FOUR BIOETHICAL PRINCIPLES

| AUTONOMY |
| BENEFICENCE |
| NON-MALEFICENCE |
| JUSTICE |

INFORM

THE FIVE PRINCIPLES OF THE ETHICAL CHÓROS

RELATIONAL AUTONOMY

Respecting the patient's separateness and independent functioning

Supporting the capacity to manage the dialectic between the demands of self-definition and of relatedness

PSYCHOANALYTIC BENEFICENCE

Enhancing the patient's capacity to mentalise

Stimulating curiosity about the unconscious inner world of phantasy and of object relationships

Facilitating integration of split-off parts of the self

PSYCHOANALYTIC NON-MALEFICENCE

Harm of misrecognition

Harm of physical impingement

Harm of non-accountability

Epistemic harm

JUSTICE

Ethical use of the imagination (i.e., imagining other people)

Monitoring of unconscious biases and prejudices

Epistemic injustice

Assuming responsibility for harm(s): the value of recognition and repair

VERACITY

The 'absence of forgetfulness'

Establishing epistemic trust

Fig. 3.1 Psychoanalytic Ethics

to avoid valorizing independence or self-reliance at the expense of relational support and connectedness to others. Personal autonomy can only emerge through the individual's dependence on others. This is a conceptualization of autonomy that is more consistent with an object relational psychoanalytic model of the mind (the model I espouse) and specifically with Sidney Blatt's two-polarities theory of personality, which has also influenced my work. According to this theory, adaptive personality development involves a capacity to manage the dialectic between the demands of self-definition and of relatedness (Luyten & Blatt, 2013). In this model, health or adaptation is characterized by the possibility to function independently while also accepting the need for others.

Autonomy has been variously defined and it is beyond the scope of this chapter to review this vast literature. Nevertheless, several definitions emphasize two features of autonomy that I want to draw attention to and examine through a psychoanalytic lens, namely 'understanding' and the 'absence of controlling influences'. Traditionally in bioethics, a person is deemed to have the capacity to autonomously choose if and only if she has at her disposal knowledge of all the 'facts' relevant to the decision and the possible consequences for her of the potential decisions (Savulescu, 1994). Many of the decisions we face in our lives and that trigger the request for therapy, for example, deciding whether to undergo cosmetic surgery, requires access to and understanding of information about the medical risks associated with this decision but it also requires an understanding of the personal relevance of these risks for a given individual. 'Understanding', as I use the term here, is thus not restricted to cognitive understanding of medical facts, but also involves self-understanding, which we would all recognize amounts to more than an intellectual understanding. Self-understanding, as conceptualized psychoanalytically, promotes autonomy through bringing to the fore 'controlling influences' so as to expand our awareness of the unconscious determinants of our decisions (Lemma and Savulescu, 2021). By 'controlling influences' I have in mind, for example, the impact of family and/or cultural pressures that are implicitly operating on our mind. We must also consider the control exerted unconsciously by repetitive patterns in our relationships with others and in relation to one's 'self', through the process of unconscious identification, that may continue to dominate an individual due to his life experiences and psychic defence structures.

Psychoanalysis thus adds to an understanding of the principle of autonomy for two reasons. First, because it subscribes to the existence of the unconscious, which subverts any simplistic appellation to autonomy as the outcome of a purely conscious rational process of deliberation about what is best for us. Second, due to its emphasis on the constituent nature of early attachment relationships, it brings into focus how autonomy is dependent on a prior condition of heteronomy. These psychoanalytic contributions lead to a richer conception of our ethical focus on relational autonomy. They challenge the primacy accorded in many strands of bioethics to a notion of a patient primarily acting in relation to his own choices, deliberations, and reasonings, while underlining the importance for the patient of questioning what he is to do with the conditions and relations that have formed him. In this model, it is the process of self-exploration (including of the unconscious mind) that is potentially transformative, liberating, and enhancing of autonomy.

Underpinning the ethical priority of respecting and supporting relational autonomy is thus my presumption that we are heteronomous *and* autonomous beings. Neglect of the interpersonal conditions within which we all develop, and within which the analytic process itself unfolds, can ultimately harm the intrapersonal constituents of autonomy. For example, denying our need for support from others can compromise the psychological resilience necessary for us to expand the range of possibilities for self-determination. In other words, having a realistic notion of our vulnerabilities and limitations, as well as possibilities, is crucial to autonomy and is a core component of the process of developing a mind of one's own. The work we do with our patients through our understanding of the transference, for example, is fundamentally connected to autonomy. Autonomy is enhanced by consideration of the implicit relational and affective templates that shape our experience of who we are and who we may feel that we *ought* to be. I am suggesting therefore that analytic work supports the development and consolidation of the patient's autonomy through the exploration of the conflicts mobilized by relatedness as they manifest in the transference relationship, and beyond it.

From a psychoanalytic vantage point, it's clear that our ability to know ourselves fully is always hedged. An undivided, all-knowing self is an overdemanding requirement for determining autonomy. Divided, unconscious motives complicate the process between decision and action. We would mostly recognize that we can believe and endorse egosyntonic but harmful conceptions of ourselves. The perceptual as well as social constituents of our identity often function as an unconscious backdrop to our sense of self and practical agency, thus eluding voluntary choice and insight. In other words, self-knowledge that is conducive to autonomy relies on acknowledging *epistemic fallibility*: we might have views about our preferences, character, and values, but we might also ignore—consciously or otherwise—inconsistencies, contradictions, and ulterior motives. Crucially both therapist and patient are susceptible to epistemic fallibility.

The final facet we need to consider with respect to autonomy is what it means psychoanalytically in an applied sense to respect the patient's autonomy in our work. There are two scenarios to consider. First, with respect to our interventions. For example, when a patient asks us a personal question about whether we have children or if we are married, and we choose to stay silent and wait for his elaboration, we need to consider whether this intervention respects or undermines the patient's autonomy. I am not suggesting that we should answer the patient's question. But if we respond simply with silence or with a question that turns the focus to potential hidden meaning, we need to consider if such a standard analytic response is equally helpful to all patients. For example, a patient who has no knowledge of the psychoanalytic method and of why such questions are not answered directly might not be able to make use of such an intervention in a way that benefits him. We must consider how our interventions do not impact patients equally.[15] At the time that we completed the

---

[15] We need to keep in mind that not all patients belong to the WEIRD demographic (Western, Educated, Industrialized, Rich, Democratic) (Henrich, 2020).

work on the psychoanalytic competences that I referred to earlier, we also put together a 'patient information leaflet' that explained, with a light touch, how a psychoanalytic therapist specifically works, and we addressed the rationale behind why such a therapist would not answer personal questions.[16] This leaflet was reviewed by National Health Service (NHS) psychotherapy service users who gave important feedback: they wished they had been able to access this kind of explanation prior to starting a psychoanalytic process, which they felt was never explained to them. One patient who had no familiarity with psychoanalysis told me that they had not returned following their assessment in an NHS psychotherapy department because the therapist refused to answer any questions about the therapy and only made interpretations. This patient could not understand why this was so and felt unable to return. Not answering personal questions, with most patients, is the most helpful approach to supporting the elaboration of the unconscious but providing at the outset some minimal orientation to why we do what we do is essential to making it possible for the patient to exercise his autonomy and meaningfully consent to a psychoanalytic approach.

Second, as I flagged up earlier, respecting autonomy involves monitoring how the patient's exploration of his life choices or the development of his personality during an analytic process may be implicitly steered by our values. We need to acknowledge this inevitable impact and rein in this tendency, as much as we can, if we want to allow the patient to use us as freely as possible to arrive at his understanding of what is best for him, considering the unconscious drivers for his choices. It is the accent on the unconscious (both the patient's and the therapist's), because it is so central to autonomy, that is the ethical priority in our work.

---

[16] The leaflet, which was written for patients accessing Dynamic Interpersonal Therapy via the NHS, can be downloaded from: https://www.ucl.ac.uk/pals/sites/pals/files/migrated-files/DIT_service_user_information.pdf.

Beneficence

So far, I have focused on the extent to which it is essential to question what we do and what we don't do in our relationship with the patient to establish if it respects his independence, separateness, and self-determination in the context of the notion of relational autonomy. You will recall that the principle of beneficence, to which we now turn, is not just about avoiding harm but is also focused on how to benefit the patient and promote his welfare. More specifically, doing good is thought of as doing what is best for the patient, that is it concerns what it means to benefit a *particular* person.

Three foci support the development of the patient's understanding of his mind. I suggest that these foci distil what it means *psychoanalytically* to 'do good' for the patient. I am sketching these in broad brush strokes but, in practice, they always need to be considered with the patient's specificity in mind. In presenting these to you, I am clear that they expose my values and biases about what I consider contributes to a 'good' life and how psychoanalytic help supports this. Divergent views about the good life will accordingly inform how other therapists and patients understand beneficence and will conceive of the aims of an analytic process. The ethical requirement for each of us therefore does not concern adherence to a specific analytic model, but the articulation of our working model does matter so that it is explicit and informs what the patient is invited to consent to.

The three foci I single out are unified by what they deliver to the patient when things go well, namely *epistemic goods*, that is knowledge derived from a lived experience in the analytic process of the workings of his conscious and unconscious mind and how it impacts his current life. When I use the term 'knowledge', I am using it therefore to denote experiential and intellectual knowledge since the analytic process proceeds along parallel lines of process and content.

First, we work to enhance the patient's capacity to mentalize,[17] by which I mean helping the patient to consider conscious and

---

[17] I emphasize that enhancing the capacity to mentalize is important, but this should not be equated with a specific brand of therapy—it describes a *general aim* that can be supported

unconscious thoughts and feelings in others and in himself in a flexible but realistic way that gives him the best chance to establish relationships that are sustaining to him and to make decisions about his life that are best for him. Constituting an authentic autonomous self is an active, dialogical, and reciprocal process. Dialogue with others facilitates reflection on our personal thoughts, feelings, and values through the interpretive lens of others, so that our subjective reflections about ourselves take on an objective and practical reality and significance.

Second, and this is a further specifically object-relational elaboration of the emphasis on mentalizing, we support the patient's autonomous functioning through the stimulation of the patient's *curiosity* about his internal world of object relationships and how this implicitly informs current functioning. A core aim of therapy is to encourage the patient's own curiosity, his 'epistemic desire' (Inan, 2012: 285),[18] that is the desire to know and to understand about his unconscious mind and to gain new experiences that challenge—even disrupt—the patient's psychic status quo. Protecting and enhancing the capacity in the patient to know himself more comprehensively requires an ongoing effort by the therapist to help the patient to mentalize.

Third, we facilitate awareness of how the patient may need to 'not know' about some parts of his own mind (i.e. for defensive reasons) and we support the (re)integration of split-off parts of the self. This is a process of restitution that helps the patient to come to terms with the actual impossibility of 'getting rid' of parts of himself and supports their reintegration so that he can be more fully himself and make informed choices from a more authentic position in himself.

In summary, the three foci of psychoanalytic beneficence are in the service of helping the patient to gain a fuller understanding of the impact of the unconscious, and specifically of internalized object relations and of his defences, on his autonomous functioning.

---

through different kinds of therapy. What matters to the position that I am outlining here, is that supporting the capacity to mentalize rests on a respect for the patient's separateness.

[18] This is a philosophical paper and Inan is not discussing psychoanalysis, but I found this term helpful for our purposes.

This process helps the patient to transform 'ghosts' into 'ancestors', as Loewald (1960: 248–249) so aptly put it. We all have a developmental history and a current life: both need to be understood if we are to understand ourselves, our relationships, and the decisions we make in our lives. Our developmental history is relevant to self-understanding because our early attachments contribute to relationship templates that are often implicit and that continue to shape behaviour in the present. This internal world of relationships gives texture and colour to each new situation that we encounter in the present: meanings and unconscious fantasies shape behaviour, thinking and feeling whether, or not, they are the originators of the behaviour, thought, or feeling. In this sense, doing psychoanalytic 'good' for the patient involves working to elaborate the internal world of object relations to extend the range of options open to the patient to make his life go better. Of course, different psychoanalytic traditions will elaborate this 'work' differently. I am merely wishing to illustrate how we might understand beneficence within the object-relational model I espouse.

The dialogical process that supports the three foci isn't only one-way: in the consulting room, the use of language implies a constant reciprocal movement between social world and individual and between patient and therapist. The value to the patient of what he can learn from the analytic encounter depends on the integrity of this process. A fundamental ethical task for the therapist is therefore to create and safeguard the conditions in which the patient's curiosity about his mind can flourish and to examine how her interventions support or inhibit this aim. The therapist's 'safeguarding' activity, in this sense, is part of the ethical labour. It emphasizes the importance of our assiduous attention to our own mind, our wishes, desires, and needs to minimize impingements on the patient. This means that we must attend to our failures of mentalizing—at times triggered by work with the patient, but not only—which can lead us to mis-recognize the patient and impinge on his mind through projective processes.

One distinctive quality of epistemic goods is that their value to the patient rests on the integrity of their facilitator or provider, in this case the therapist. If the information that is provided or elaborated through the dialogue is false, contaminated by the values of the therapist without due acknowledgement, or manipulated in the service of meeting the needs of the therapist, this undermines the chances for establishing *epistemic trust*. This refers to 'the disposition of a person to accept and trust that the information of other persons is authentic, trustworthy, generalizable and relevant to the self' (Knapen, et al., 2022: 313). The establishment of epistemic trust is what facilitates the 'learning' that arises out of the analytic encounter and ensures that it stands a better chance of generalizing beyond the confines of the consulting room.

Non-maleficence

If we work to the psychoanalytic *telos* of helping the patient to develop a mind of his own through 'using' the analytic relationship, as I have been suggesting, then follow four core forms of harm that we can perpetrate (*maleficence*) and that we must work hard to avoid. This list is not intended to be exhaustive and represents my attempts to date to conceptualize harms in the context of psychoanalytic work.

The harm of misrecognition
The first is the *harm of misrecognition*. This results from our failure to relate to the patient as an intentional thinking and feeling being with both conscious and unconscious desires, hopes, and fears that are *separate to our own* and that have legitimacy by virtue of their source, that is they emanate from the patient as partial knower of his own self. Partiality is not a function of being a patient and being unwell; as I have repeatedly emphasized, it is a property that all of us share given that we can only ever be partial knowers because we cannot anticipate the as-yet-unelaborated unconscious.

One way to harm people is precisely to harm them in their capacity as knowers and as epistemic agents. When we attribute to the patient intentions, feelings, or thoughts that are not his own, or we fail to recognize intentions, feelings, or thoughts that are his own, we perpetrate a form of harm and injustice. At its best, analytic listening and the interpretations that derive from it, lays the foundation of autonomous functioning—we become autonomous agents partly through being recognized by others as intentional beings. When we fail to appreciate the importance of the patient's narrative and give it legitimacy (which is not the same as 'believing' the patient or 'privileging' his narrative), and we assert our 'expert arrogance' (Harcourt, 2021: 733), we perpetrate a harm. My choice of the word 'arrogance' may strike a provocative chord. Much of the time I am sure that we would not recognize what we do as being arrogant. But when we become married to certain ideas or ways of doing analytic therapy, and we do not expose ourselves to the corrective that comes from the patient, or simply from another perspective, we are being arrogant. We are of course entitled to having a point of view, but rarely is a helpful point of view one that does not yield to engagement with other voices and resists all challenge. Even so, and as I will return to in Chapter 5, there will be analytic relationships, as in life, where the difference of opinion cannot be constructively elaborated.

Recognition is a fundamental human need. The German philosopher and sociologist Axel Honneth's (2005) theory of recognition, drawing on the object-relations theories of Winnicott and the work of Jessica Benjamin, speaks to the shared human need to be recognized.[19] To become an autonomous ethical agent in the modern world, he argues, we must enjoy self-confidence, self-respect, and self-esteem, each of which requires, for its development, a distinct kind of recognition. Recognition is important, according to Honneth, because the formation of ethical personhood depends on it: it is key to identity development for all of us.[20] We do not become

---

[19] A disciple of Jürgen Habermas, Honneth constructed a moral sociological theory of human suffering. He recognized three spheres of human recognition: love, legal recognition, and social esteem respectively. Each type of recognition is linked to a shared norm, a positive relation to self, and specific patterns of social interaction in which recognition is sought and granted—or not.

[20] The importance of social recognition beyond the immediate family is now receiving due attention. See, for example, Luyten et al.:

> . . . research on disadvantaged individuals clearly demonstrates that the experience of a broader social context that fails to recognize the individual as a person—that is, that fails to mentalize the needs of that individual to belong and be part of a

ethical subjects by some monological process of internal development; we become so by engaging in interactions with others and learning to see ourselves through the perspectives that others have taken on us.

According to Honneth, characteristic forms of disrespect or misrecognition may be observed. This occurs when the shared norms governing recognition are violated. Such denials of recognition not only result in shame and anger but also hold the potential to inflict psychic damage because misrecognition, he writes:

> '. . . represents an injustice not simply because it harms subjects or restricts their freedom to act, but because it injures them with regard to the positive understanding of themselves that they have acquired intersubjectively'. (Honneth, 2005: 131)

Honneth's emphasis on the intersubjective context in which we come to understand ourselves is well placed and relevant to our work. It sensitizes us to why our interventions are so critically important: they can make a fundamental difference to how the patient becomes intelligible to himself and whether this understanding facilitates his development in a direction that is congruent with what he values or whether it undermines autonomous development through imposing the therapist's interpretations and values.

'Recognizing' the patient in the context of our work begins with the acknowledgment that we cannot know in any absolute sense the mind of the patient (i.e. mental states are opaque). Although we can sometimes make accurate guesses about what the patient may be feeling or thinking, they are no more than informed guesses that may or may not lead to an understanding that the patient will deem helpful. Importantly these are *our* ideas, which we must clearly mark as such. To say that our knowing, at best, is uncertain, as we saw in Chapter 1, is not to suggest that we should claim to erase knowing. Our theories and dynamic formulations of the patient have a place,

---

community—lies at the heart of feelings of loneliness, alienation, and estrangement, leaving these individuals vulnerable to psychopathology. (2022: 21)

but they cannot be upheld to be always more correct or truthful than the patient's. Questioning how we relate to our theories and how they can potentially harm the patient is part of working ethically.

Therapist and patient may well disagree. I am not advocating a mirroring process that confirms what the patient wants to hear or can tolerate hearing or suggesting. I believe there are risks in positioning ourselves only or primarily as mirrors or soothing objects; marking our separateness and challenging the patient are essential to the patient's development. Rather, I am emphasizing the importance of marking our interventions as reflecting our own thoughts and not as having de facto superior epistemic value than the patient's own understanding of his own mind. Theories or formulations that are clung to rigidly can perpetrate a form of normative violence as we assign specific roles or pathologies to the patient, constructing the patient according to the authority of the therapist. A most painful example of this normative violence has been the (now predominantly historical) pathologizing of homosexuality by psychoanalytic practitioners.

The harm of physical impingement

The second type of harm is the *harm of physical impingement*. An experience of misrecognition, as I have been discussing, typically results in an impingement because the patient is not related to as a separate subject. However, the specific harm of impingement, as I define it here, results from a breach of the *physical* boundary between therapist and patient, which always also involves a mental breach given that body and mind are irreducibly connected. It is conceptually and clinically valuable to single out the specific harm of physical impingements in the context of the analytic relationship because of the body's central organizing role in our functioning and sense of who we are. It is not just that intrusions into the patient's body by the therapist through sexual boundary violations invariably betray misrecognition of the patient and of his separateness, and involve a deep (I would say, irreparable) breach of trust (even if transferentially the patient may desire the intimacy). It is also because the body is the point of meeting and integration between a person's subjectivity and the objective world, such that physical and sexual transgressions also infringe on a basic and universal right to *bodily integrity*.

It is precisely because the body is the medium through which we interact with others, and it is core to how we execute our agency, that we have such a wide-ranging right over our own body. As Herring and Wall (2017) emphasize, it is the right 'to exclude' and the decision 'to include' that give the value to touching that is wanted and desired: physical interactions, touches, and exchanges gain their value and meaning largely through being chosen and valued by the individual. A sexual transgression is therefore always an impingement on the patent's bodily integrity and not just on their bodily autonomy. *Bodily autonomy* protects a person's capacity to make his or her own decisions in relation to their body. The right to bodily integrity is conceptually different. It refers to the right to exclude all others from the body, which enables a person to experience his body as intact and free from unbidden physical interference. The use by the therapist of the body of the patient, in the specific context of a treatment that actively uses the analytic relationship to help the patient, and that claims to understand the vicissitudes of this relationship because it subscribes to a notion of the unconscious, is therefore wrong at an exceptional level.

Epistemic harm

The third harm is *epistemic harm*. When we take on the role of 'psychoanalytic therapist' based on the specialist training that we have undertaken, we assume certain responsibilities as an epistemic authority in this specific domain. Our specialist knowledge and skill in facilitating the exploration of the unconscious is our 'added value' to a prospective patient, or else he would be best advised to talk to his neighbour or friend about his problems. These non-professional conversations may turn out to be helpful—they might possibly be even more helpful than seeing a therapist. However, I am simply stating the obvious: the role of therapist communicates to the patient an 'added value' and this, I suggest, is our psychoanalytic knowledge about the mind and about the analytic process, which are the epistemic goods that we provide and instantiate through how we use the analytic relationship, and that distinguish us. Importantly, this specialist knowledge is dialogic: it is not just that we have some general psychoanalytic knowledge about the mind, but we also have a uniquely psychoanalytic appreciation of how some of the knowledge that will be relevant to the patient is an emergent property of the analytic interaction itself (Felman, 1982). In other words, we are not imparting ready-made knowledge; rather we are creating a new condition for knowledge: the creation of an original learning disposition because we learn through a specific orientation to the other. This places us in a position of significant responsibility: many people who seek therapy are epistemically 'hungry' (Luyten et al., 2022: 22) and this may amplify the attendant risk of 'epistemic credulity' (Luyten et al., 2022: 22).

We are profoundly dependent on one another for epistemic goods:[21] for truthful information about the world, for understanding complex topics, and for understanding our mind. These dependencies make us vulnerable to manipulation from knowledge bearers (e.g. therapists, doctors, teachers) and those who disseminate knowledge (e.g. media) and who may abuse their epistemic authority. As a putative expert, a therapist can manipulate or misrepresent the patient's state of mind, or she can withhold information from a patient or fail to give information that could help the patient to understand the analytic process. For instance, as I mentioned earlier, for a patient who has no prior knowledge of how psychotherapy works, a classical analytic non-response by the therapist to a question such as whether she has children[22] or about the process itself without sharing any account of the purpose of this non-response, deprives the patient of information that he may need to orient himself to the therapy and to make an informed choice about whether to engage

---

[21] Watson (2018) has emphasized the notion of 'epistemic rights', that is rights to epistemic goods such as knowledge, understanding, information, and truth, the right to withhold information, and the right to privacy. Epistemic rights comprise a complex set of entitlements that provide justification for the performance and prohibition of certain actions regarding epistemic goods.

[22] To be clear again, I am not suggesting that the therapist should answer the question about children, but that she needs to offer the patient an explanation of why she may choose not to answer so as to make more transparent to the patient the process that she is trying to establish, and that to the best of her knowledge, will help him.

with the therapy. Or if we think back to the days when homosexuality was viewed by many psychoanalysts as a form of pathology, we now regard the therapist as giving the patient misinformation based on prejudice. In the analytic encounter therefore, we can harm the patient in his capacity as a knower of his mind and as a decision maker.

The *harm of non-accountability*

The fourth harm is the *harm of non-accountability.* If we are all capable of harming our patients, at least some of the time, we add to the harm if we are then unable to assume responsibility for it and be accountable, by which I mean specifically that we fail to mark the event (e.g. a moment of distraction or a critical edge in our tone) and do not acknowledge its harmful impact as such. In other words, mentalizing is necessary to ethical practice but not sufficient. We can imagine a therapist who is very good at mentalizing, recognizes her errors to herself and/or in supervision, but does not act on this recognition with the patient, perhaps because admitting the error shames her (Crastnopol, 2019). When we transgress in some way, we commit one kind error or violation but, as Levin points out, '. . . the deeper, *ethical* failure' (2010: 78) is when we don't acknowledge what happened and explore this with the patient.

As in everyday life, if we make a mistake that adversely impacts another person, we acknowledge that we have made a mistake and so take responsibility for how this may have impacted them. Failing to take responsibility for our mistakes (which includes hiding behind one-way conceptualizations of notions such as 'enactment' where the patient is the one who is seen to 'invite' us to respond in a particular manner) is therefore a form of harm. We will return in more detail in Chapter 6 to the corresponding 'Duty of Candour'.

Justice

I have been discussing the analytic process unfolding between therapist and patient and to which each party brings to bear their respective internal world of object relations. We also need to recognize that both participants in this process are always embedded in a very specific socio-cultural, political, and historical moment that informs their respective internal and external realities and the analytic process itself, introducing prejudices and biases that, in turn, can introduce unfairness. The most profound sense of justice, in my view, refers to what Scarry (1998) singles out as the ethical necessity of 'imagining other persons'. Being just or fair in the analytic dyad relies on the ethical use of our imagination, '... placing ourselves in the space of mental "Otherness"' (Scarry, 1998: 46), divesting ourselves of our 'idols' so that we can see how the world looks from another vantage point.[23] The respect for otherness and the receptivity to what feels foreign to us so that we can then welcome this otherness into our mind, are essential anchors of 'just' practice. Hosting otherness and difference in our mind is one of the most challenging requirements of our work.

I want to draw attention to three principal ways in which we can perpetrate injustice as psychoanalytic therapists. In different ways these forms of injustice reflect the operation of *unconscious biases and prejudices*, and hence require that we are alert to how our ways of responding to our patients may be profoundly shaped by implicit values and assumptions. Essentialist views about gender or sexual desire, for example, have shaped public history, our individual histories and psychoanalytic theories. As therapists, even though our psychoanalytic brief, as it were, is the internal world, we still have a responsibility to understand how these external facts impact our patients and our own mind and therefore cannot be neatly parcelled out from an understanding of the patient's internal world.

First, as we saw in Chapter 2, considerations of justice require us to always keep an eye on the external world to ensure that the services we offer are fair and accessible. This invites us to consider how we

---

[23] In ethics, Rawls' (1973) 'veil of ignorance' is often invoked to arrive at just decisions. Rawls encouraged us to approach decisions from the standpoint of ignorance about our actual position in the world (for example, our genetics, our wealth) and to imagine what decisions we would make if we could not be guaranteed what we know about who we are, what privileges we have, or what needs we might have across the lifespan.

might need to modify the provision of psychoanalytic therapy to help specific patient groups or to make it more inclusive. A good illustration of this issue is the transition to online interventions triggered by the Covid-19 pandemic in 2020. This worldwide event focused our discipline's attention on how a modification of the setting could make psychoanalytic therapy more accessible to more people during a time when in person meetings were difficult and travel was restricted all over the world but also during a time when the demand for psychotherapy increased dramatically. Prior to the pandemic, prejudice precluded an open engagement with the potential merits of such a medium (Lemma and Caparrotta, 2014). We might say that the concern about diluting the gold of psychoanalysis and preserving a mode of delivery that was familiar, and perhaps even suited a particular generation of psychoanalysts (including my own generation), precluded a calibrated and just examination—that is, in its own right, and not triggered by the exigencies of a pandemic—of how we could help more people whose socio-economic or geographic circumstances prevented them from accessing psychoanalysis as we believed it should be practiced.

This is not to suggest that online therapy is functionally equivalent to in-person therapy. This is not a view I share (Lemma, 2017). My point is merely that online therapy has something to offer that is of value and part of its value resides in its accessibility, that this is question of justice—amongst others—and that prior to the pandemic, many within our discipline displayed prejudiced positions on this rather than questioning how modifications of the setting might be ethically required to ensure fair access to a form of intervention that we deem to be helpful. However, even my point about the merits of accessibility requires further qualification. Moving to online work may exaggerate inequality of access for those on the wrong side of the digital divide either because they don't have access to a computer or to a space within their home in which they can safely have therapy. The debate about online therapy is thus a very good example of the complexity of ethics and of the requirement to balance competing principles: solely advocating the merits of online work may ignore justice considerations as much as dismissing its value.

A second form of injustice that we need to monitor is *epistemic injustice*,[24] that is when an individual's communications are under-valued in communicative practices, a position that has been elo-quently articulated by Miranda Fricker (2007). Fricker focuses on the unjust ways that we distribute credibility, in what she calls the 'credibility economy'. She draws attention to how social resources such as knowledge and expert authority are distributed unequally between different groups 'with the upshot that some social groups are unable to dissent from distorted understandings of their so-cial experiences' (Fricker, 2011: 39). For example, Jeremy Clarke (2019), in a notably rare application of the concept in a psychoana-lytic paper, reframes Freud's account of Dora's story as an example of epistemic injustice, where he argues that Dora's credibility—by virtue of being a woman—is undermined due to her hermeneutic marginalization.

When we systematically exclude people of a particular social identity, such as women, or people with mental health problems, and many intersectional identities, Fricker suggests that we effec-tively embargo or diminish various ways of knowing. For example, when we do not treat 'lived experience' as a criterion of credibility, or we ignore a patient's narrative because they are 'psychotic', we exclude knowers who deploy those ways of knowing. And when knowers are excluded for epistemically defective reasons, Fricker suggests that this causes and contributes to epistemic oppression.

Just as the patient may be invested for defensive reasons in var-ious kinds of 'unknowing', so too the therapist. Mason (2011) notes not only that marginalized people may lack the hermeneutical re-sources to understand their own experiences or oppression but also that those in dominant social groups may remain ignorant of

---

[24] According to Fricker there are two forms of epistemic injustice: testimonial injustice and hermeneutical injustice. Testimonial injustice occurs when the level of credibility attributed to a speaker's word is reduced by prejudice operative in the hearer's judgement, while hermeneu-tical injustice results when testimonial injustice is so persistent and socially patterned (as any-thing driven by prejudice is likely to be), that it contributes to hermeneutical marginalization, 'That is to say, it will tend to create and sustain a situation in which some social groups have less than a fair crack at contributing to the shared pool of concepts and interpretive tropes that we use to make generally share-able sense of our social experiences' (Fricker, 2016: 4).

the oppression of marginalized groups. As Mason puts it, these two types of unknowing are:

> . . . an unknowing to which members of nondominant social groups are subject by virtue of their systematic hermeneutical marginalization and an unknowing to which members of dominant groups are subject by virtue of their ethically bad knowledge practices. (2011: 295)

While it's certainly important to focus on how marginalized persons are harmed by lacking access to hermeneutical resources to help them understand their own experiences, Mason reminds us that one way that structural oppression maintains itself is by dominant group members also not knowing about the systems of oppression in which they operate, participate, and perpetuate (even unintentionally). In turn, this raises an interesting question, namely do we as therapists have a moral *duty of inquiry*? In professional contexts, such as medicine and psychotherapy, it is clear that holding certain mistaken beliefs poses a threat to the well-being of others. Therapists who held (and a few still hold) a view that homosexuality was a pathology were perpetrating harm. They held such beliefs based on prejudice and small group samples of selected patients who made it onto the couch, as it were. As a professional, when we label any behaviour as a pathology, this is a form of action—and an exercise of power—that has serious, potentially harmful consequences for those so labelled. In this sense we could claim that the obligation to inform oneself beyond the narrow confines of our own discipline has clear ethical grounds: it diminishes the possibility of harm by broadening our knowledge base thereby reducing the risk of prejudiced positions. And yet, most therapists have undergone psychoanalytic trainings in which the contributions of other disciplines (not least research) to bring in other perspectives are not routinely introduced and robustly engaged with. Clearly, it would be essential to articulate with greater specification when and why a moral duty of inquiry obtains, even if we agreed that it is relevant—I am merely introducing the idea here to highlight how thinking about ethics has a broad reach inviting not only individual introspection but also challenging institutional training efforts (see Chapter 8).

The notion of epistemic injustice encourages us to take note and question not just our own listening but also the extent to which our institutions can become more receptive to listening to what they may well not want to hear. In the related fields of psychology, psychiatry, and sociology we find a substantive and growing literature on the notion of epistemic injustice. It is striking that a concept that is so central to any endeavour that relies on listening to another person's narrative and responding to it, such as psychoanalytic work, has only featured seven times in published psychoanalytic papers, the earliest of which was only published in 2019—the paper by Clarke to which I have just referred.[25] I underline this observation because it points to how we are late in the day in engaging with this concept and reveals that we have given limited conceptual space to understanding how the therapist, through her *potentially* totalizing knowledge, may discredit the patient as an epistemic agent.

I have emphasized the value of the concept of epistemic injustice. This does not imply that it is therefore unproblematic. A significant challenge arises when the concept is invoked to justify privileging 'lived experience' as the ultimate reference point in an understanding of a patient's predicament—this is what is referred to as 'epistemological privileging'. The patient's narrative is, of course, fundamentally important but this does not mean that it is therefore always the truth and that the psychoanalytic interpretation is the oppressive narrative. Conviction about 'what happened to me' or strongly held feelings about our wishes or anxieties cannot be the final arbiter of what is true. Likewise, for psychoanalytic convictions about what is 'normal' or 'psychopathology'. Expert knowledge-production should be open to scrutiny, but the patient or 'experts by experience',[26] do not have an inviolable epistemological privilege. The value of the

---

[25] Pep-web articles word search on 21 July 22.
[26] This is a term used to describe people who have personal experience of using or caring for someone who uses mental health and/or social care services.

notion of epistemic injustice lies in its function as a cautionary concept that alerts us to the way that knowledge is not evenly distributed and that understanding (ours and that of the patient) is at best partial and evolving (see also Chapter 1). The patient's 'lived experience' must be the starting point of a process of understanding but it cannot exhaust our understanding of the patient's mind in its complexity.

The third sense of justice that is relevant to the analytic encounter, and that overlaps with the principle of veracity (see Section 5), is that justice requires us to be truthful about how we can and do harm our patients. Justice, in this sense, refers to a cycle of *recognition* and *repair*. Here I am deeply indebted to the work of Jessica Benjamin who has emphasized how the experience of being recognized is integral to the possibility for repair. Benjamin powerfully captures this in her discussion of the 'moral third', which refers to

> . . . the values, rules and principles of interaction that we rely upon in our efforts to create and restore the space for each partner in the dyad to engage in thinking, feeling, acting or responding rather than merely reacting (2009: 442)

According to Benjamin, this sets the conditions necessary for repair, noting 'the lawfulness involved in repair':

> . . . lawfulness begins 'primordially' with the sense that the world offers recognition, accommodation and predictable expectations and develops into truthfulness and respect for the other, and faith in the process of recognition. (Benjamin, 2009: 442)

In referring to lawfulness, Benjamin has in mind a very particular quality of lawfulness, that is law as the importance of (re)establishing symmetry or harmony after a rupture. It is a vital feature of a 'just' world and she underlines the 'order' that is re-established through the experience of being recognized by the other. This, she suggests, can only occur if we are prepared to take responsibility for our contribution to an impasse or when we make an error:

> When we as analysts resist the inevitability of hurting the other—when we dissociate bumping into their bruises or jabbing them while stitching them up, and, of course, when we deny locking into their projective processes with the unfailing accuracy of our own—we are bound to get stuck in complementary twoness . . . the principle of reciprocal influence in interaction, [which] makes possible both responsible action and freely given recognition. (2004: 10–11)

Recognition here means being mobilized by the situation to turn towards it rather than away from it; it is also a first step towards 'acknowledgement' in the sense of taking responsibility for harm we might have done, or been implicated in. The experience of being recognized provides an opportunity for restoring a sense of a 'we'[27] that re-establishes epistemic trust as the patient experiences the therapist's movement from relating to herself and her needs towards a relationship with him with due recognition of his experience and needs. We will return to these themes in Chapters 5 and 6.

Veracity: The absence of forgetfulness

Finally, I want to introduce a fifth principle: *veracity*. Veracity is not always considered to be a separate ethical principle even though it is highly relevant to ethics. For example, Beauchamp and Childress (2013) view veracity as a specification of the other principles such as autonomy or justice. I present it here in the psychoanalytic ethics model I am outlining as an *absolute* ethical principle and independent obligation that ranks in importance with autonomy, beneficence, nonmaleficence, and justice. To respect the patient's autonomy, and to maximize benefit to the patient, to limit harm and to be just, the therapist must also be truthful and keep the psychoanalytic promise (see Chapter 1). A promise is only as good as the

---

[27] Joe Higgins (2020) specifically discusses a 'we-mode' that '(. . .) emphasises the relational 'we' character of thinking and acting with others (2020: 804).

integrity of the person who makes it, which is why the commitment to being truthful is a *sine qua non* of ethical practice.

My penchant for etymology led me to search for the ancient Greek word for truth, which is *a-leitheia*. This a word made up of two components: *ἀ* (ah) = 'absence of' and *λήθη* (*leithei*) = 'forgetfulness'. The etymological root thus exposes an important meaning of 'truth'. If we think about truth as the 'absence of forgetfulness' we are anchored in the ethical importance of remembering what has happened or is happening (i.e. what has gone wrong)—the etymology thus links veracity to a form of *witnessing*. It is as vital to witness and to remember what has happened historically in society, as it is in the context of the history of our everyday encounters with our patients in our consulting rooms. I choose for our purposes the definition of truth as the 'absence of forgetfulness' because it places a necessary emphasis on the ethical importance of 'not forgetting', that is of taking responsibility for our actions, past, present, and future and of explicitly acknowledging them. It reminds us of our part in exposing and bearing witness to the truth of what transpires in all our interactions.

In the context of psychoanalytic work, veracity deserves to be singled out given that truth in psychoanalysis is foundational. The treatment is based on the patient who is invited to tell the truth and the therapist who must be trustworthy given that the patient, by entering the analytic relationship, is exposed to the risks inherent to any relationship of dependency. The therapist's truthfulness is a constant pillar as she tries to balance competing ethical demands, but we are always at risk of succumbing to our shared tendency towards self-deception. We are well versed in the baleful effects of self-deception and denial and monitor these tendencies in our patients, but we also need to be on the alert to such tendencies in ourselves, not least when things go wrong in the analytic relationship. The analytic process is ethically compromised unless the therapist can also be truthful about the process and its risks, and about the contributions that she makes to this process, for better and for worse.

Truth is important because as therapists we are striving to establish trust between us and the patient so that the patient can relax his epistemic vigilance and make use of the interpersonal opportunity for learning that a trustworthy analytic relationship can offer. 'Relevance theory' (Sperber and Wilson, 1986; Walaszewska and Piskorska, 2012) proposes that the perceived 'relevance' of what another person offers to us is determined by the extent to which we feel we are in a relationship with someone who relates to us as an agent with a valid subjective experience worthy of engagement. The aim of all communication, including in the analytic dyad, is to generate *epistemic trust* (Fonagy et al., 2019), so as to foster an individual's willingness to consider new knowledge from another person as trustworthy, generalizable, and relevant to the self. Epistemic trust makes it more likely that the patient can use what the therapist offers at the level of both content and process to safely challenge and potentially change his way of thinking and feeling. Insights and lessons learnt from the interpersonal experiences that emerge within the analytic exchange, and that are perceived by the patient to be truthful, makes them worth having, that is they can be 'used' by the patient to challenge himself and to learn something new about how he functions in the world. None of this is possible if we are not truthful about the impact of our contributions to the process—we will return to this in Chapters 5 and 6.

To be truthful, we must acknowledge that our professional lives are not only conditioned by our developmental histories and other important demographics. They are also shot through with unconscious desires and libidinal investments and governed by the imperative to rid ourselves, through projection, of that for which we may not yet be ready to take responsibility. Being truthful requires us to be prepared to examine the psychic investments and values embedded in our clinical decisions and interventions. Remaining open to feeling and thinking about what is happening between us and the patient such that we can rigorously analyse those investments is part of the ethical labour. This, as we have seen, involves living in the complexity of one's life and adhering to the truth of that complexity—a truth that involves assuming responsibility for the way one's desires and psychic investments inform that irreducible complexity and inevitably impact on the patient.

4
The Ethics of Analytic Listening

I believe we have seriously underestimated the foundational role of ethics in psychoanalysis because to consider it seriously inevitably trains the lens on us as individuals in relation to our patients.

—(Kite, 2016: 1153)

The analytic relationship is unique in offering permissiveness of discourse: the therapist listens but does not impose restraint or judgement. Listening is the cornerstone of analytic technique, and it is a highly complex activity. 'Complex' because listening requires attending to multiple levels of meaning and intentionality, that of the patient's unconscious and conscious utterances, that of the therapist's conscious and unconscious utterances, and finally at the level of the intersubjective matrix where therapist and patient meet and create a unique interaction determined by both parties. We listen to what may not yet have been thought about and/or verbalized. This means that we listen out for the backstory to every conscious narrative. At its best, the analytic encounter legitimizes the fact that the patient always has more to tell, and the therapist can only facilitate this if she is prepared to listen to her own backstory mindful that she invariably communicates more than she knows. The five principles that I set out in Chapter 3 are the ones against which we can ethically evaluate how we listen to the patient.

To listen in this very attuned manner to the unconscious, Freud set out the spine of what is referred to as the analytic attitude. The analytic attitude describes the therapist's position or state of mind in relation to the work. This state of mind—as the group of expert clinicians representing different psychoanalytic traditions concurred when we carried out the work on psychoanalytic competences—is characterized by receptiveness to the patient's unconscious communications and to the unfolding of the transference (Lemma et al., 2008). The therapist's state of mind functions as 'the keeper of the analytic process' (Calef and Weinschel, 1980) and so protects the privileged space that is the analytic encounter. Nowadays there is no consensually held notion of shared technique, such that even definitions of the analytic stance are subject to variation across different schools of psychoanalysis. Notwithstanding such variation, three features of the analytic stance are typically agreed on, namely neutrality, abstinence, and anonymity (Freud, 1912a; 1913). In many respects these describe how to minimize impingements on the patient's space for exploration and for how he can 'use' us, not least those intrusions arising from the therapist's needs. Although they have traditionally been conceptualized as a part of technique, I suggest that these three concepts represent the earliest formulations of ethical precepts concerned with protecting the use that the patient can make of the therapist (see also Pinsky, 2017). However, to get an in-depth grasp of the ethical labour demanded of the therapist as she listens to her patient, we are rewarded when we go beyond psychoanalysis and turn to the work of the French philosopher, Emmanuel Levinas, whose phenomenology of otherness is challenging and thought-provoking. His ideas have entered psychoanalytic thinking in North America, Israel, and Europe but he remains a relatively neglected figure in mainstream British psychoanalytic thinking, though there are a few notable exceptions in this respect (e.g. Frosh, 2011; Frosh and Baraitser, 2003; Black, 2021).

Levinas and preparedness for the other

We not only need to focus on listening to the patient but we must also listen to *how* we listen. The therapist's personal equation filters how we listen. All too often, we hear only what we can apprehend in ourselves but there is so much that we miss altogether or only partially hear. If, as I suggested earlier, we accept that (a) the analytic relationship is bidirectional, (b) the therapist not only reacts to but also acts on the patient's experience, for better and for worse, and (c) the therapist bears asymmetrical responsibility for what transpires between her and the patient, then it follows that the act of listening necessarily engages us in an ethical process in relation to the patient. This is why listening is more than just a technique: it is, as Elizabeth Corpt puts it, a 'responsibility' (2018: 223).

Because we use ourselves to do our work, we are confronted from the outset with an ethical challenge. Listening is demanding because '. . . to listen is to situate oneself in such a way as to be able to take in the otherness of the other' (Corpt, 2018: 222). This availability to the other and in service of the other reaches far beyond anything that could be meaningfully described as technique. Several key contributions to the ethics of the psychoanalytic encounter draw on Levinas' (1969) foundational precept that responsibility for the Other defines ethics, most notably the work of Chetrit-Vatine (2014), to which I will return, but first I want to introduce you to some of Levinas' core ideas.

In *Totality and Infinity* (1969), Levinas maintains that ethical obligation cannot be objectively grounded in a rational system of laws but results instead from recognition of the otherness of the Other. Crucially, Levinas argues for the priority of heteronomy (i.e. the determination of the subject by another) over autonomy (i.e. self-determination). Reversing the more standard privileging of autonomy over heteronomy, Levinas articulates a distinctive and ethically demanding relational emphasis in his theorizing of responsibility:

> I speak of responsibility as the essential, primary, and fundamental structure of subjectivity. For I describe subjectivity in ethical terms . . . the very node of the subjective is knotted in ethics understood as responsibility. (Levinas, 1985: 95)

For Levinas, heteronomy is the state of subjection to the Other. Levinas's whole project is an attempt to unsettle our tendency towards what he refers to as 'totalising' ways of thinking, challenging the complacency of the self-sufficient 'I'. An example of such totalizing knowledge might be when we categorize patients, lock them into diagnostic labels and justify our clinical decisions based on the diagnoses as if they related to undisputed 'facts'. Yet, what is required of us, Levinas argues, is to question the so-called facts:

> The justification of a fact consists in lifting from it its character of being a fact, accomplished, past, and hence irrevocable, which as such obstructs our spontaneity. (1969: 82)

'Facts' or what we take to be 'facts' such as the specific psychoanalytic theories that orient us to how we listen, thus potentially impede unencumbered receptivity to what the patient tells us. Instead of spontaneity, we encounter the patient through the filter of what we expect to be the 'normal' resolution of the Oedipus Complex, for example. Levinas essentially invites us to consider how knowledge is a form of power that we can deploy in ways that potentially harm the Other.

Rather than being a subject who chooses, autonomously, to accept responsibility for others, Levinas argues that we are responsible for and to the other person before we are capable of choice, that is, we only become a subject in heteronomy. This has important implications for how he understands moral obligation. Moral consciousness, for Levinas, is not an experience of our values but refers to an access to Otherness, and this Otherness he names *visage* (the face). The ethical is the location of a point of alterity—or exteriority— which cannot be reduced to what Levinas refers to, by contrast, as 'the Same'. Otherness is witnessed in the 'face' of the person looking at me. In the face-to-face relation, my natural narcissism is interrupted, and I find myself provoked to respond to the Other with responsibility: '. . . the face summons me to my obligations and judges me' (Levinas, 1969: 215). The face thereby plays a dialogical role: 'face and discourse are tied' (Levinas, 1985: 87). Its presence disrupts me from my narcissism (Butler, 2006) and calls me to respond in such a way that I am in essence held 'hostage':

> I am pledged to the other without any possibility of abdication. I cannot slip away from the face of the other in its nakedness . . .; to approach is to be the guardian of one's brother; to be the guardian of one's brother is to be his hostage. (Levinas 1998: 71–72)

His philosophy thus places centrepiece the problem of the normative status of the other, or if you prefer, of the 'ought' of ethics. The Levinasian ethical choice is essentially to welcome the 'stranger' in the Other and '. . . to share his world' (Wild, 1969: 14).

'Why does the other concern me?', asks Levinas, 'Am I my brother's keeper?'. These questions have meaning only if one has already supposed that the ego is concerned only with itself, is only a concern for itself' (Levinas, 1986: 106). For Levinas, such an orientation can never provide the basis for a meaningful ethics. In a world that priorities the self's ego, others are experienced as impediments on the road to self-actualization, wherein 'every other would be only a limitation that invites war, domination, precaution' (Levinas, 1986: 108). Put simply, ethics is not ethical when it is geared towards the pursuit of self-actualization, when my interests are prioritized over the interests of the Other.

Responsibility for the Other is asymmetrical, in Levinas' sense. By this he means that I have no right to demand from the Other what the Other has a right to demand from me (Atterton, 2007). My responsibility for the Other is therefore not contingent on the Other construing his duty towards me in a reciprocal manner. This presumption is core to his philosophy:

> The intersubjective relationship is a non-symmetrical relationship. In this sense I am responsible for the other without waiting for reciprocity . . . reciprocity is his affair. (Levinas, 1981: 98)

Levinas's view is one of 'radical responsibility' in so far as he stresses that the responsibility for the Other should not preoccupy itself with what the Other is with respect to me, that is, what the Other can provide for me but only with the fact that the Other is the one *I* am responsible for, someone *I* must look at and look after. This Other makes a demand simply by virtue of his existence. In this respect, the Other presents a demand on 'me', interferes with 'my' sense of liberty and freedom, and calls on a responsibility that I cannot refuse. Because being responsible for the Other does not entail reciprocity, it exposes the asymmetry in the relationship; it exists simply as an ethical imperative, as that which makes us human. Indeed, Levinas makes it clear that this relationship of responsibility—the ethical relation—is primary, rather than following from something pre-existent. For Levinas, the human subject does not first exist and then engages in ethical relations; rather, ethics is the defining feature of subjectivity itself. More specifically, it is our acceptance of the moral demands of responsibility that makes us the unique individuals that we are.[1] It is in this sense that moral responsibility precedes the ontological self: we become a human being only through acceptance of moral responsibility. A refusal to do so makes us less than fully human.

Phenomenologists, with whom Levinas identified early on in his career, grappled with the problem of Otherness, but Levinas grew dissatisfied with how this was conceptualized in Western ontology in general. According to Levinas, such understandings missed a crucial point, namely the way that the Other summons us. In other words, the Other's need does not have to be uttered in order for me to feel the summons *implicit* in the Other's presence. The summons is binding. In this encounter with the Other, the duty to respond to the Other abrogates my drive to protect my self-survival. And it is here that Levinas strikes a deeply familiar psychoanalytic chord that is also the spine of ethics: the ethical relation to the Other stems 'from the fact that the self cannot survive by itself alone, cannot find meaning within its own being-in-the-world, within the ontology of sameness' (1986: 24). This is the core of the intersubjective life that

---

[1] See also the Danish moral philosopher, Knud Løgstrup (2020) whose notion of the 'ethical demand' resonates with Levinas' philosophy.

Levinas prioritized, and which constitutes the central locus for his ethics. This is deeply relevant to our work.

In this all too brief overview of Levinas' philosophy, I hope that I have nevertheless conveyed how his thought adds depth to our attempt to understand why listening is so 'complex'. Responsible listening depends on an act of generosity, suspending our world with all its familiar and contingent assumptions to welcome a potentially disorienting and destabilizing otherness. Levinas' articulation of responsibility also makes clear why analytic work, as I have been suggesting, is specifically an ethical labour because it squarely focuses on the unconditional—even traumatic—demand imposed on us by the Other (McCoy Brooks, 2013). This exposes the reality of our 'impossible profession' (Freud, 1937)—its very impossibility resulting from a demand that we cannot escape from but from which we are always, to varying degrees, trying to divest ourselves.

Chetrit-Vatine's (2014) seminal psychoanalytic text on ethics is deeply rooted in Levinas' thought. A key basic premise in her thinking is that the therapist must understand that the analytic relationship is at once both seductive and ethical. She argues that the analytic situation, much like the baby's primal situation, is a repository of 'ethical seduction'—what she refers to as the 'double asymmetry in the analytic situation'. The seduction requires a sensitive attunement by the therapist to what is demanded of her as a matter of course:

> . . . the origin of ethics as responsibility for the other resides in his or her potential capacity to let him or herself be touched, penetrated, taken hostage, interpellated by the other's fragility. (2014: 163)

These claims on the therapist's mind cannot but solicit at times the need to push back, to resist the experience of being taken over, to be 'taken hostage', as Chetrit-Vatine vividly describes it following Levinas, because the patient's otherness reminds us of the 'ought'. Chetrit-Vatine understands this in terms of her notion of the 'matricial space transference':

... [it] is a non-linear transference. It is not reproduction. It refers not so much to what has taken place or what has partially taken place, but to what ought to have taken place. (2014: 95)

Not all patients have experienced trauma or some form of deprivation in childhood that results in the experience in the transference of the kind of 'ought' that Chetrit-Vatine has in mind. However, she reminds us that especially where this has been the case, but not only then what is needed from the therapist far exceeds the conscious contract of therapy. Unless we understand what the patient needs, we may be either seduced into thinking we can deliver this demand or feel imposed on by it—either way we fail the patient. In this sense, we might say that 'the ethical relation is not a mutual enterprise . . ., but an unconditional surrender to the suffering of the patient' (McCoy Brooks, 2013: 94). As we look at the face of the Other, Levinas urges us to take in the vulnerability of that Other, the precariousness of the Other's life. The 'face' confronts us with an unpalatable truth: we become aware of our capacity to cause pain to the other, of our potential for violence (Butler, 2012). How can we understand this? Stephen Frosh applies himself to this very question as he observes that the apprehension of the Other's demand in the context of what he calls 'reciprocal vulnerability' mobilizes in each of us '. . . something elemental, in the sense of foundational and therefore shared, both in precariousness and in violence' (Frosh, 2015: 386).

I have suggested so far that the essence of ethical listening involves preparedness for the Other, and this otherness, always demands something that conflicts with the therapist's desire[2] and narcissism. The Other primarily demands space in our mind. This is what the therapist promises to offer the patient but even in the best of circumstances, at some stage, she will fall short of this promise. This is because narcissism is a permanent feature of being human. The potential for iatrogenic effects is therefore significant, no matter how much personal therapy/analysis we have undertaken. We must

---

[2] Desire is used here to refer both to the therapist's sexual desire and to their non-sexual desires (see Chapter 1).

contain and detoxify our own personal excesses, and this is an on-going, life-long process.

Levinas' emphasis on the one-directional nature of responsibility for the Other, brings into sharp focus how the therapist's own needs and desires cannot but be thwarted at every turn given that she cannot expect anything from the patient: no gratitude, no getting better, no gratifications of any kind.[3] To describe the therapeutic exchange in these terms confronts us with why the work is so demanding and why it should not surprise us that enactments and ethical breaches occur all too frequently, and that this possibility is not reserved for a small group of therapists quite different from 'us'. As I discuss in Chapter 5, ethical breaches and errors of different kinds are not the exception—they are far more commonplace than we like to think. The good-enough therapist is not the one who manages to avoid making errors. Rather, it is the one who expects this to be the case, some of the time, and works actively within herself, and with the patient where appropriate, to take responsibility for what happens when things go wrong:

> ... If the therapist does not take refuge in the convenience of considering his experience to be the result of projective identification, then he has gained some purchase on his desire. The analytic process can proceed, then, relatively unburdened by the confusion of self and other. (Wilson, 2013: 471)

But to do this, the therapist must also know about her *hatred* for the work (see also Chapter 1). As John Steiner cautioned, 'I suspect that what analysts must struggle with is that their love for psychoanalysis coexists with a hatred of it' (2000: 642). Along similar lines, Nathan Kravis (2013) claims that 'hatred of analysis is a normative experience for the working clinical therapist' (2013: 89). He argues that this acknowledgment is necessary to sustain the onerous demands

---

[3] This is not to suggest that we don't hope that our patients will be helped by us and feel able to express gratitude—perhaps in itself a sign of development for particular patients—but we cannot expect it and resent the patient if he does not get better or express gratitude.

that analytic work imposes on the therapist. He underlines the narcissistic deprivation that the therapist is subjected to contemporaneously with the need to come to terms with her fallibility. This accounts for the feelings of shame, inadequacy, and of fraudulence that bedevil us. As if matters were not complicated enough, Pinsky (2011) shrewdly observes that self-effacement carries its own ethical risks because 'self-effacement, too, can become a form of self-idealization' (Pinsky, 2011: 368). Whichever way we try to square it within ourselves, our narcissism is here to stay, and humility may simply turn out to be a cover-up.

Reciprocal ethicality

It will be evident by now that I am drawn to Levinas' work and deem him essential reading. Even so, he has also rightly been challenged as elaborating an 'extreme ethics' (Rozmarin, 2007: 327) that is not only personally challenging but also requires some qualification in order for us to integrate it into how we understand and approach the analytic encounter. The psychoanalytic dialogue, and the type of listening that it calls us to engage in, cannot be conceived as a one-way street, as we saw in Chapter 1. I have focused so far primarily on the therapist's resistance to taking the patient into her mind because this is one of my primary concerns in this book. However, we cannot ignore that the resistance to otherness is also operative in the patient to varying degrees. In some patients the difficulty in tolerating otherness is a central presenting feature in the work and can manifest in a refusal to accept the therapist's separateness and a difficulty in working within the analytic boundaries. Acknowledging this reality introduces much needed nuance to any discussion of responsibility in the analytic encounter. At its best, an important feature of the analytic relationship is perhaps most usefully conceived as mobilizing a reciprocal ethicality, as Eyal Rozmarin suggests or promoting 'ethical equality', as Robert Drozek (2019: 194) puts it. It is precisely the hallmark of the unique ethical nature of a psychoanalytic process that, as Rozmarin puts it, the 'other deserves a hearing' (i.e. *both* parties):

Psychoanalysis cannot put one ahead of the other, nor the other ahead of me. It can give voice to the one, then to the other, in a dialectic that has no resolution, only the continuous establishment of a relationship where both can live. This is why life, when viewed through psychoanalytic discourse and practice, can be neither a story of self-realization, nor a story of dedication. It can only be a conversation, a relation among these stories or positions. And for life as conversation or relation, psychoanalysis can serve, again in a minor way, as both reasonable and ethical model. (Rozmarin, 2007: 359)

Rozmarin's account resonates personally but it is essential to keep in view that in this 'conversation', responsibility when things go wrong nevertheless resides first and foremost with the therapist. By this I mean that given the 'psychoanalytic promise', if I as the therapist cannot take you (my patient) into my mind, or I use you instead of allowing you to use me, within the bounds of the analytic contract, then I, as the therapist, have to take responsibility for this happening between us even though you (the patient) may have also, or even mostly, contributed to it.

As we listen to the patient, we will sometimes face a breakdown between the patient's and our version(s) of reality. For example, say a patient calls out what he perceives to be the therapist's emotional absence. We can imagine that in some instances the patient may well have perceived an 'absence' because of the activation of an internal model of the absent object, perhaps provoked by an upcoming break (a marker of the reality that the therapist does indeed withdraw from the patient during her break), rather than in response to an actual withdrawal by the therapist in the session because she is preoccupied with her own needs. In the best of circumstances, this experience of the therapist then becomes a focal point for exploration, comparing respective versions of reality in a manner that neither denies the patient's version nor defers to it. In other words, just as we need to consider the risks of not taking responsibility for our mistakes, there is also a potential risk if we don't address the patient's and therapist's subjective divergences for what they are: differences of understanding or opinion that might reveal something of value. Here, I suggest, the ethical stance is to respect difference and to acknowledge that this may well be experienced by the patient as hurtful, perhaps even as intentional (i.e. as the therapist perpetrating harm because she does not espouse the patient's view), but this keenly felt subjective reality does not necessarily make it a fact in external reality. How this is taken up in an interpretation will vary depending on preferred technique.

I have returned to some of the questions that were touched on in Chapter 1 because they are central to understanding our responsibility towards the patient. Acknowledging reciprocal influence or our epistemic fallibility as we listen and then interpret, does not necessitate adopting the postmodern position that there is therefore no truth—a complex and ongoing debate that I cannot enter here. Suffice to say that analytic work requires recognition that any process that seeks to get to the truth calls on both participants to elaborate their version of it. At times both parties will need to be prepared to take different, yet respectful, positions towards the understandings that evolve. If something goes wrong along the journey towards this truth-seeking, we take responsibility in so far as we are responsible for truthfully engaging with how this could have happened. Our responsibility is to listen respectfully and non-defensively in the service of understanding what went wrong from the patient's perspective and what part, if any, we may have played in this. To put it plainly, 'if it happens on my watch, then I have to look at the part I *may* have played in this system and take care of the patient'. 'Taking care' always involves a commitment to trying to understand what has happened in the analytic relationship. Even when we can determine that, to the best of our knowledge, we did not materially contribute to the patient's subjective experience that we have caused him pain or harmed him in some way, we remain the responsible party to ensure the patient's confrontation with his internal objects is addressed with due care.

All intimate relationships, including the analytic one, are perhaps best conceptualized as a work-in-progress. *How* we listen to each other contributes to this evolution. Over time different iterations of narratives and affective experiences are elaborated. These are shaped by the respective idiosyncratic psychic contingencies of each party (e.g. their unconscious world of object relations, their developmental histories). This process involves two subjectivities but the unconscious intrapsychic configurations that inform the unfolding of a particular dynamic cannot be assumed to always be equal in their force and impact on the dyad at a given point in time. Therefore, there is a place for a therapist's interpretations of what may be happening in the analytic dyad. This is because there will be times when the therapist is better placed than the patient (given the unconscious pulls that the patient may be in the grip of at a given moment in time) to have a perspective on what is happening. This does not mean that the therapist's account is always right, but only that at a given intersection she may be able to hear something as she listens to the patient, which the patient cannot yet discern in himself, because in that moment the therapist is not psychically overtaken by the same dynamic pull operating within the patient. Of course, this cuts both ways. Even so, our personal therapy, training, supervision, and the cultivation of the *ethical chóros*, are all ways of limiting our intrusion into the patient's space such that we can bring 'something more' to the patient's exploration of himself than a conversation with a friend. If we cannot be expected to be at least potentially able to be more alert to our blind spots than the patient, at least more of the time, then this begs the question: what is our added value?

Obstacles to listening: The pedestrian and equestrian approaches to analytic listening

To listen well enough, we must approach the task with the expectation that this intention (i.e. to listen well enough) will always be subverted and that it is incumbent on us to be aware of the obstacles that interfere with listening.[4] There are as many obstacles as there are

---

[4] Parts of this section also appear in Lemma (2013).

anxieties and defences so I cannot pretend here to address this question in any exhaustive manner. In Chapter 1, I have already highlighted how unmentalized desire and hate can create many obstacles to listening and hence to ethical practice.

If the patient as Other always demands too much, this inevitably places pressure on the therapist to mute what the patient is saying. This is likely to interfere with the therapist's capacity to listen. Our internal obstacles to listening will be variously determined by our respective vulnerabilities, conflicts, and theoretical and/or institutional allegiances. But we cannot ignore that sometimes it is our tenacious relationship with selected psychoanalytic theories that creates the obstacle to listening. Theories give us sustenance and/or feed our narcissism and they can also get in the way of listening. The comforts they offer are significantly offset by the risk they potentially introduce to our capacity to listen to the patient. I was vividly reminded of this when some years ago now, a talented colleague began one of our supervision sessions with an apology: "I'm afraid that what I said to the patient was really quite pedestrian. I know I should have taken up the transference but instead I asked the patient a question. I know this was wrong". Even before I could question this assumed 'wrong', she went on: "I have been thinking about what made me do this. I think this patient finds it hard to think and I get caught up in this and end up asking inane questions". When I hear this kind of statement, I am curious both about what may have indeed been going on between the patient and the therapist (was this an enactment, for example) *and/or* about what may be going on between the therapist and psychoanalysis as an object in her mind, that is, in this case, her transference to the concept of working in the transference—an instance of Bacon's 'idols of the cave' (see 'Introduction').

The demands made on us by the very nature of our work may help us to understand the fierce attachments we can develop to ideas. We feel the need for an organizing structure in the face of a patient's pain. At times the burden of responsibility may be (unhelpfully) sidestepped through allegiance to theoretical belief systems that act as a kind of intellectual protection racket. Under this kind of pressure and needing to manage the challenge of 'not knowing', we can find ourselves relating to our theoretical ideas and techniques not as guiding principles but as fetishes (Denis, 2008; Ferro, 2009). As we all learn through the reality of work in the consulting room, analytic work requires the relinquishment of a magical investment in any one theory or technique at our disposal. Such unexamined attachments often interfere with our capacity to listen to the patient and to take responsibility for him in the sense that I have been discussing so far. Ethical practice requires that we be prepared to question these attachments.

To return to the previous supervision session: as my colleague and I reflected on her intervention it became clear that her anxiety about not 'doing the right thing' had interfered with her capacity to listen to the patient's response. Her confessed 'sin', as I listened to her, struck me as a simple but well-timed clarificatory question in the context of the patient's report of a difficult exchange with a work colleague, which promoted a deepening of this patient's exploration of the event. It helped this patient to stop and take notice of what was happening in the 'here-and-now' of his affective experience as he was relating this event.

When my colleague apologized for her intervention, I was intrigued by her choice of word to capture her anticipation of how I would view her intervention: she feared that I would find it 'pedestrian'. From the Latin *pedester* meaning 'prosaic or plain', something pedestrian is the mark of something, de facto, unremarkable, or unelevated. In Latin, *pedester* is contrasted with *equester* which means 'on horseback', (i.e. elevated)—a presence that is noticeable: one even must 'look up' to see the rider. Moreover, the rider benefits from an aerial view (a view, quite literally, from above) that cannot be appreciated from the busy street through which the pedestrian travels or in which he dwells.

For me, the contrast between the pedestrian view and the equestrian view captures an important feature of analytic listening that has ethical implications: as therapists we need to strike the right balance between immersion in the analytic field where both patient and therapist are working together, 'on the street', as it were, maintaining the horizontal relationship, whilst also retaining an 'aerial' view so that we can think with the patient about what is happening on the street. The aerial view is indispensable but it also requires us to monitor that the view it affords us is not shared with the patient from an 'on-high', superior position. This latter position is consequently riskier and may tip the analytic relationship into malignant verticality (see Chapter1).

I imagine I am not entirely alone in finding myself, sometimes for extended periods of time, silently 'walking on the street' with the patient, or getting lost, or misreading the signposts or, at best, making pithy interventions that function a bit like punctuations of the journey along the way. The feature they share is that they are 'unremarkable' (the pedestrian view), that is, they do not offer to the patient the therapist's more saturated processing of what is being revealed in the psychic landscape (the 'aerial view'). The latter would be more of a 'this is what I think is happening in your mind now' type interpretation, which can all too easily slip into a dangerous 'this is this is what I *know* is happening in your mind now'. It is interesting to consider what can be gained if one is simply a pedestrian, walking along the street with the patient. By this I mean using our interventions to accompany the patient along the sidewalk of his associations, or to create crossings to the possibility of representing experience or making the kind of 'behind the bar' observations that Bolognini (2005) has so evocatively written about.

As Bion (1962) articulated, K as a 'getting to know' (Ogden, 2004) can readily become an internal imperative to know *the* answer. The function of interpretation in the service of enlivening curiosity, of opening a dialogue to support the development of the patient's autonomy, becomes hijacked by 'knowing that', rather than being used in the service of engaging the patient in a 'process of knowing' about his mind (Bell, 2011; Busch, 2010), which is essential if 'doing good' for the patient involves helping him to mentalize (see Chapter 3). Knowing, Levinas points out, '. . . becomes knowing of a fact only if it is at the same time critical, if it puts itself into question, goes back beyond its origin' (1969: 82). Knowing, for Levinas, is an open-ended state of mind that seeks to gather information and questions the very process of seeking as much as it questions the facts thus gained.

At its best psychoanalytic listening is an enhanced form of recognition and of witnessing[5] (Reis, 2009) by virtue of its emphasis on unconscious mentation. If we can speak of the ethics of psychoanalytic listening, I suggest that it approximates a commitment to a form of *unsaturated* listening that allows the therapist to 'return' something that belongs to the patient so that he can hear himself say what he has known all along but has not yet articulated. This 'return' supports autonomy, as I argued in Chapter 3. I refer to this as an ethics of listening because it is predicated on what the patient needs (i.e. what is best for him) and not what the therapist wants or needs as she makes an interpretation (e.g. to please her supervisor or to fit in with her idealized version of being a Kleinian or a Freudian). If this might be the essence of an ethics of listening, then an ethical interpretation based on this form of listening would be an expression of a K relationship with the patient to support the patient's capacity to experience and know himself as someone who has a mind. This type of listening, and the interventions that flow from it, are rooted in a respect for the otherness of the Other, which requires a commitment to remembering two cardinal technical rules that, I suggest, keep us on the ethical side of practice, namely (a) being mindful of the fundamental opacity of mental states (the patient's and our own given the existence of an unconscious mind to which we are not privy) and (b) ensuring that we 'mark' our interventions, that is we signal that we are sharing *our* thoughts and that these are not the final word on what the patient may be thinking or feeling.

---

[5] Over the last 20 years, some therapists have drawn specific attention to the importance of another very particular type of listening, namely *witnessing*. The term is used in at least two ways and as such causes some confusion. In the first sense, witnessing denotes silent but active presence 'engaged non-intrusiveness'—listening in a way that is not seeking what can be interpreted (Poland, 2000: 21). It refers therefore to a type of listening that does not seek to do '. . . anything more active about it' (1998: 21). The second use of witnessing denotes a clearly active form of listening that is explicitly linked to ethics in so far as Boulanger (2012), for example, argues that clinicians are 'morally obligated' (2012: 318) to bear witness when an external event has caused so much disruption to the patient's sense of self that a witness is necessary to validate the extent of the psychic distress.

5
On Getting it Wrong

Ever tried. Ever failed. No matter. Try again. Fail again. Fail better.

(Samuel Beckett, 1983: 13)

If my patients read this book, there will be some who will say that sometimes I get things wrong and misunderstand them and that this has caused them pain. They are right. I have thoughts about what those evaluations of me mean in the context of the transferential relationship with a given patient over time but I don't want to dwell on that here because that is not the point of this chapter and, in any case, such transferential formulations—even if correct—do not invalidate the fact of my errors in some cases. Like any therapist, I do get it wrong. When we get something wrong within the range of reasonable expectations of what we can offer as therapists,[1] and within the parameters of the ethical framework I set out in previous chapters, first and foremost we need to recognize what has happened and take responsibility for this. This stands, I suggest, no matter what specific meaning it might hold in a particular interaction and how we might understand it psychoanalytically.

Writing a book about ethics does not right the mistakes I have made in the past nor does it immunize me against making mistakes

---

[1] This specification is important because there are limits to what we can offer and unless we are clear about these limits, we can set up unrealistic expectations, which can confuse the patient.

in the future but it helps me to have a clearer place in my mind for what I ought to do such that the next time round, as Beckett puts it, even if I might 'fail' again, I hopefully 'fail better'. I use 'ought' advisedly because this is a moral imperative that can steer us towards better practice as long as it does not give way to a 'Super'ego (Bion, 1962), that is an ego destructive superego 'ought' mandate. This latter is a primitive superego that results from early splitting and needs to be differentiated from the normal superego:

> The abnormal superego usurps the status and authority of a normal superego and entices the ego to turn away from life, to dissociate itself from its objects and ultimately to destroy itself. (O'Shaughnessy, 1999: 861)

Enthrallment to 'Super'ego driven moralism is a tipping point for ethical breaches because one form it can take is to seductively elevate the self by encouraging thinking that relegates ethical breaches to being the exception rather than the rule, only committed by a small group of colleagues regarded as 'other'—Dimen's (2011) 'rotten apples'. It protects us from awareness of our own flaws and encourages us to look at the fallen colleague from 'on high'. Therein lie the twin dangers of narcissistic self-soothing and moral triumph: 'I am not like that', or 'I was better analysed', or 'I had a more in-depth training' than the person who is exposed as the 'rotten apple'.

Taking up the moral high ground puts us in a dangerous place in our mind. In this respect, the research on moral self-licensing is sobering. It illustrates that because good deeds make people feel secure in their moral self-regard, they are then more likely to be less vigilant. For example, when people are confident that their past behaviour demonstrates compassion, generosity, or a lack of prejudice, they are more likely to act in morally dubious ways without fear of feeling heartless, selfish, or bigoted (Merritt et al., 2010). To put it bluntly, when we feel that we have already contributed to something good, this seemingly frees us to behave badly (Monin and Miller, 2001). Splitting, as we recognize psychoanalytically, pays short-term narcissistic dividends but comes with significant ethical costs. Indeed, the research on moral hypocrisy[2] testifies to the all too human tendency to hold double standards and exposes the pernicious impact of this split. It reveals how we consider ourselves to be morally responsible when we are asked about it, but in practice studies suggest that this is a 'surface appearance of morality' (Batson et al., 1997: 1346) and our behaviour often betrays self-interest and minimization of the 'wrong' in our behaviour.

Taking seriously the impact of our errors requires us first to take our work seriously: a psychoanalytic intervention is a very powerful intervention. Just as an insight can be transformative, an interpretation about the patient's mind that is coloured by a therapist's own projections can be deeply harmful. We simply don't do justice to the enormous skill required to enter another person's mind and hence the responsibility that ensues. Although (mostly) our patients don't die if we get something wrong, we can still do significant harm. We must take ourselves seriously if we are to take seriously what can go wrong in our work. Approaching our errors requires us to first conceptualize how we 'do wrong' by our patients and then identify the occupational risks that expose psychoanalytic therapists specifically to 'getting it wrong'. This is the focus of this chapter. In Chapter 6, I will then address how we can constructively respond to our mistakes and thus honour the Duty of Candour (DOC).

On getting it wrong

Types of 'wrongness'

Ethical vulnerability lies at the core of the psychoanalytic profession. Unless we grasp the ubiquity of errors, we expose our patients to risk. I use the term 'error'—not at all an ideal word but

---

[2] Batson et al. define this as the state of mind in which 'Morality is extolled—even enacted—not with an eye to producing a good and right outcome but in order to appear moral yet still benefit oneself' (1997: 1335).

it's the most expedient—to denote the overall category of 'when things go wrong'. This can cover, for example, misjudgements (e.g. taking into our practice a patient who cannot make use of psychoanalytic therapy), lapses in attention (e.g. distraction, forgetting), or moments of misattunement. In the sense that I have been using 'ethics', all of these instances would represent ethical incidents. I reserve the term 'violation' to describe actual physical and/or sexual transgressions and sustained emotional abuse of the patient to meet the therapist's own needs. Overall, I have in mind therefore not just the most egregious ethical breaches but also our functioning at sub-optimal standards, for example because we may have taken on too much work at a given point in time, our focus is compromised, and we cannot avail our mind fully during the agreed session time to understanding the patient's mind. This represents a breach of our 'psychoanalytic promise' (see Chapter 1). Even though this most likely would not reach a regulatory threshold for action against a therapist, such breaches are no less important and deserve scrutiny.

My focus on how we can get it wrong does not mean that the patient's subjective experience is the final arbiter. I am not ignoring those instances when the therapist may have indeed done her best, yet the patient may disagree and feel he has been let down or neglected and consider that the therapist has not acted in his best interests. Repetitions in the transference with an object felt to be rejecting or neglectful can contribute to painful and challenging impasses, which in turn can mobilize defensiveness in the therapist. In such instances, whilst we would not consider the resultant impasse to be caused by therapist error, it is nevertheless important for the therapist to take responsibility for how she manages her response to a challenging patient who may need to control or denigrate her and acknowledge how her responses may amplify the impasse. That said, in this chapter I am working on the assumption that we have made an error in the service of reflecting on how we can understand the nature of our errors, the risks we are exposed to, and use this as the basis for thinking about how we respond once we have made an error.

It is helpful to differentiate different categories of error, of which there are at least three broad types, hence this list is by no means intended to be exhaustive.

- Technique-based errors (e.g. delivery of an interpretation at the wrong time or in a manner that is evidently critical of the patient; inappropriate therapist self-disclosure).
- Clinical judgement-based errors (e.g. mishandling of a child protection issue following a disclosure in a session, failing to act on an assessment of clinical risk).
- Normative errors (e.g. violation of a code of conduct).

No matter the nature of the error, the definition of when something has 'gone wrong' reflects that it is so because:

The therapist has a duty to the patient.

↓

This duty is breached.

↓

The patient is harmed.

↓

The harm is caused by the breach of that duty.

From an ethical point of view, any type of error can compromise the ethics of care, which are the foundation of our work. I am deliberately not focusing in detail on whether some wrongs are 'more wrong' than others in any absolute sense (i.e. their relative moral weight) or whether they meet criteria that would instigate a formal investigation by a registering body. As I hope will be clear by now, I am as interested in embedding and supporting the *ethical chóros* in the therapist's mind as a routine practice to engage us in monitoring our work more systematically and doing our best for patients, as I am in breaches that lead to being struck off a professional register.

However, and self-evidently, the nature of the error is significant. We cannot equate the impact of a sexual boundary violation and the exploitation this represents (Burka et al., 2019) to a temporary lapse in our attention to what the patient is saying because, say, we are worried about a personal family matter. Our self-interest is at play in that moment too, and impinges on the patient's space, but it is not *exploitative*[3] of the patient in the way that a sexual violation is. It would be exploitative if such lapses were recurrent and essentially the therapist was being paid for *not* listening to the patient. However, and even assuming the technical or attentional lapses are not sustained, from the patient's perspective, just as in cases of an actual violation, there may be a (temporary or sustained) disruption of trust in the therapist as a 'good object' (Elise, 2015) whose duty it is to protect the analytic space in the service of the patient developing an understanding of his mind.

Within this broad category of 'getting it wrong', I distinguish two types of ethical breaches in terms of their impact on the analytic process. One that leads to *fracture*, that is it breaks the analytic relationship irreparably; the other creates a *relational gap*, which if mentalized, can potentially be transformed into an opening that adds perspective to the work of therapy. This is only possible if what has gone wrong can be reflected upon non-defensively with the patient. When occasional errors are acknowledged and reflected on, they do not typically lead to fracture. Enactments that are repetitive and unmentallized are more likely to lead to fracture.

Ethical breaches that lead to a fracture result when there is a repeated intrusion into the patient's mind by the therapist's own needs and when the patient's body boundary is crossed. As I suggested in Chapter 2, the protection of the body's integrity (i.e. the body's inviolability) is considered by many to be a basic human right (Nussbaum, 2000). Bodily integrity is not something that a person possesses as such; rather it reflects a *process* that needs protection and recognition

---

[3] Gruenberg (1995) makes the important point that exploitation can occur even if the patient is not harmed. He gives the example of a therapist who, based on information shared by a patient during a session about stocks and shares, uses this information for his own ends. Here, Gruenberg argues, the patient does not suffer direct harm but is nevertheless exploited.

from others, including the legal system. A sexual violation in the context of a relationship of dependency and power asymmetry, such as the analytic one, represents a violation of the patient's bodily integrity but it reaches far beyond it. Respecting the patient's bodily integrity is important not only because it amounts to protecting the patient's physical autonomy (i.e. what he freely chooses to do with his body) but also because body and mind cannot be separated such that a violation of the body's boundary invariably also entails a psychic intrusion. A sexual violation intrudes into the patient's imaginings and understandings of his body, its limits, and characteristics.

One important reason why the boundary of the body is inviolable, and the analytic relationship cannot recover after its breach, is specific to the nature of the analytic relationship. Psychoanalytic treatment involves a degree of regression, dependency, and safe seduction as intense feelings towards the therapist as an attachment figure are stimulated and infused with Oedipal longings. It is in the very nature of the analytic encounter that the patient exposes himself to a potentially intoxicating and destabilizing dependency, laced with erotic longings, through the relationship he develops with the therapist and that one day he must relinquish. Cutting to the chase, Adam Phillips shrewdly observes: 'Psychoanalysis is about what two people can say to each other if they agree not to have sex' (2008: 1). When things go well, this is the paradox that the therapist safeguards (Pinsky, 2014). None of this can take place safely unless the abstinent boundary set by the therapist is strictly maintained. Once this boundary is crossed, the necessary conditions of safety cannot be reclaimed again with the same therapist.

There are ethical breaches and errors then, such as a sexual boundary violation, or when there is a sustained impingement on the analytic space by the therapist's own self-interest, where the integrity of the process as well as of the therapist are irretrievably compromised because the therapist is effectively exploiting the patient to get her own needs met. Most breaches, however, are more helpfully conceived as the therapist's 'delinquencies'.[4] By this I mean, as Joyce

---

[4] Again, the sustained or one-off nature of these 'delinquencies' is key in determining the nature of the ethical breach.

Slochower, defines them: 'the virtually ubiquitous ways in which analysts deliberately withdraw from the therapeutic endeavour' (2003: 451). Research on the triggers to sexual boundary violations reveal that these are more likely when the therapist is lonely, isolated, disillusioned, or disgruntled and suffering from a narcissistic injury (Gabbard, 2017). But of course, any of these factors can also account for an emotional withdrawal from the patient that does not result in a sexual intrusion but is nevertheless impactful. The excellent paper by Slochower (2003) that addresses this question gives a fascinating insight into the range of 'delinquencies' that have been reported to her. Unlike the more obvious exploitative behaviours, the breaches detailed by Slochower illustrate a withdrawal of the therapist's attention and emotional investment in the patient's process. I am quoting her at length to give a clear sense of the panoply of behaviours this term covers:

> ... making a note to oneself about a forgotten task, adding to a grocery list, planning an event, filing or painting one's nails, combing hair, putting on makeup, surfing the web, searching a dating website, eating a snack, skimming a magazine or journal, checking email, buying airline tickets online, reading correspondence, pumping breast milk, watching a sports scoreboard online, writing patients' bills, deliberately cutting a session short by a minute or two . . . . Strikingly, in only two of these instances did patients indicate that they were aware of the therapist's breach. One person reported to me that while lying on his analyst's couch, he sniffed several times and then asked, "Do I smell nail polish?" He did. Another colleague reported that a patient's previous analyst regularly ate dinner during their sessions until one day the patient exploded with the comment, "What is this, a fucking picnic?" . . . . There is a second group of misdemeanors that are engaged in openly during face-to-face sessions, in full 'view' of patients. These include eating or taking long phone calls, using a treatment hour to discuss a matter of personal concern, asking patients to recommend physicians, stocks, discount clothing stores, restaurants, hotels, and so on. (Slochower, 2003: 453–454)

These behaviours are breaches of undisputed professional norms that are not explicitly enshrined in a code of ethics: we don't need the code to spell out that we should not be doing our manicure or eat lunch or fall asleep during a session. Even so, it clearly happens. Moreover, as Slochower notes, even when the inappropriateness of the behaviour is registered privately by the therapist, often the therapist fails to take responsibility for this and thus commits '. . . a second breach by lying or rationalizing in an effort to cover up their action' (2003: 454). However, if the therapist takes responsibility for what has happened and reflects on it within herself, or with the patient where appropriate, I suggest this kind of scenario, and the relational gap that it exposes, may nevertheless be bridgeable with some patients.

Recognizing that we get it wrong: Internal and institutional resistances

Delineating different types of errors assumes that we recognize in ourselves their possibility (hypothetically) and their occurrence when they transpire, but this is not something that we can take for granted. Intrapsychic and institutional resistances often work against open recognition of ethical breaches (Gabbard, 2015; Dimen, 2011; Slochower, 2017; Levin, 2021). Such incidents mark us, they leave their trace, as Dimen put it, and by '. . . sullying the whole, taint each of us' (2021: 68). No-one relishes being tarnished with the 'unethical' brush. This is why we may well deny or turn a blind eye to what is happening in our own work and around us in our psychoanalytic societies.

Clinical seminars during training rarely focus on when things go wrong where it is the therapist and/or our method that are under scrutiny, not the patient. Of course, clinical seminars and supervision address challenges that the therapist encounters or enactments the therapist feels drawn into, but by and large the discussion centres on a one-way street. The framing narrative is often that the patient invites the therapist into an enactment rather than on how the therapist's own limitations or personal equation may be at play. Of course, there are times when the patient is enacting a sadistic dynamic and needs to enlist the therapist into this despite the therapist's attempts to mentalize what is happening. Sometimes the patient is in the grip of a toxic abnormal superego such that malignant narcissism dominates the clinical field and defies the therapist's best efforts. My emphasis on the therapist's contribution should not be read as overlooking these kinds of scenarios. All this we know. I am focusing instead on what we may not want to know about ourselves.

If we want to minimize ethical breaches, we need to reconfigure the layout of our conceptual mapping with respect to the therapist's inevitable personal contribution to the unfolding of the analytic relationship. There are too many one-way streets. I am not suggesting that there is a functional symmetry between patient and therapist because the patient is unarguably more dependent and more vulnerable, he is the one seeking help and the therapist is not the one being analysed. In the best of circumstances, the therapist is authorized to be in that role because she has committed herself to a process of close introspection during her training and beyond it such that she should be in a better position than the patient to manage her own mind even though all interactions with another person, including with our patients, can potentially exert all manner of unconscious pulls. We are not exempt from such interpersonal dynamics but most of the time in the clinical setting, we are hopefully better able to recover from their pull and respond to them constructively. However, we need to allow the traffic, as it were, to flow both ways so that we can more clearly identify in our minds the 'two-person nature of the problem', where this is the case (see Wilson, 2013, for example). In turn, this can help us to consider constructively the 'two-person nature of the solution' (Benjamin, 2006).

You might well think that I am setting up a straw man and that all good and decent therapists readily acknowledge when things go wrong. If this were the case, then we do well to wonder why negative outcomes and dropouts remain comparatively neglected topics in the vast clinical literature on psychoanalytic therapy. Why don't we study these and write about it more? There is a paucity of published accounts of treatment failures. This does not mean that our profession is full of 'bad' therapists who are covering up their mistakes or experience of difficult endings with their patients. But the comparatively small literature on this subject might signal that we don't feel it is possible to discuss treatment failures in a supportive setting and that doing so might reflect badly on us. Yet, as I have been suggesting throughout, the reality is that we all make mistakes, we don't always function at our best, and it is unfortunately not possible to help everyone who seeks therapy. Our discipline cannot improve unless we can bear to face our limitations and failures.

When Kächele and Schachter published their paper on treatment failures in 2014, and they entered the term 'psychoanalytic failures' into Pep-Web, they found six entries. I took the liberty of repeating this search again in early 2022 and found that over the ensuing eight-year period, the psychoanalytic literature has only acquired five more entries. In their original paper they conclude:

> Psychotherapeutic and psychoanalytic failures are largely invisible to many therapists who refuse to see them. Treatment failures may be seen as threatening by many therapists who view them as undermining the effectiveness of their therapeutic role. Failure of psychotherapeutic and psychoanalytic treatment is a major clinical problem of substantial dimensions. (Kächele and Schachter, 2014: 233)

I am sure that I am not alone in contributing to the data reported by Kächele and Schachter who draw attention to the prevalence of countertransference induced failure as one of the denied aspects of psychoanalytic therapy:

> If leaving treatment prematurely and either failing to achieve therapeutic benefit or worsening of the emotional disorder are included, this probably includes 50% of all patients who initiate treatment. Of patients who initiate psychoanalytic treatment, only approximately 50% go on to reach a mutually agreed termination. (2014: 249)

Negative outcomes are by no means rare exceptions. Many of us will have seen patients who did not feel previous therapies were helpful or who report more clear abusive breaches. And some of us, and I include myself in this, will have had at least one patient who ended their therapy dissatisfied with us, feeling that it had not helped them at all or enough. I am not thinking here of instances where the patient had unrealistic expectations or took a passive role and expected to be 'fixed' or could not allow the therapist to help him because he had to undermine anything good. Rather, I have in mind here patients for whom, for example, we are not a good fit perhaps because of what they touch in us or because it is not possible to safely provide what is needed in the clinical setting in which we practice. With the benefit of hindsight, more often than not, the error is not that we agreed to take on the patient in the first place because it is not always possible to discern these dynamics or risks so clearly at the outset. The error lies in not recognizing and/or owning up to the bad fit soon enough and not being more open to the possibility that ending the therapy might have been better for the patient so that he could find a better fit. In such instances we do well to ask ourselves why we avoid ending the therapy. Is it because we need the patient? Do we need to see ourselves as being able to manage a difficult situation rather than accept our limitations or the limitations of our method? Do we focus more on the patient's pathology rather than on how we may not be the best fit for a particular patient? Of course, these are all very complex questions with which we all struggle in our professional lives. This is so because when working, say, with a patient who develops a pronounced negative transference, we might consider it to be an expected part of the work to survive and metabolize the attacks on us and on the analytic work in the service of the patient's longer-term gain. We would anticipate that this could take a long time such that it may be some years before we might take the view that the work is not progressing and conclude that to persevere with the therapy is the least ethical thing to do.

We encounter an added challenge when facing therapeutic impasses: because a central aim of therapy is to help the patient to take responsibility for himself and his actions, in some cases the patient may be unconsciously invested in attributing to the therapist the role of being the 'perpetrator' of hurt or shame and the patient is the 'victim' of cruel treatment. Where this is the case, John Steiner describes how the therapist's invitation to the patient to consider his part and responsibility is experienced by the patient.

> . . . as the analyst's denial of any responsibility for the difficulties of the analysis. Here important questions are raised that remain unresolved. How is the analyst to help the patient face responsibility when this leads inevitably to shame and guilt, feelings readily defended against by projective identification? What factors enable guilt to be bearable so that the patient's love and respect for reality can be mobilized to embark on reparation, rather than on revenge and blame? (2000: 641)

We tread a fine balance between shouldering our responsibility for an impasse and addressing the patient's contribution to it. These complicated dynamics can then make it very hard to discern when it is indicated to bring a therapy to an end. Not only are we sometimes confronted with an impasse but there are also simply limits to what we can do as a therapist. Psychotherapy is far from being a panacea for psychic pain and life's challenges. Our ethical responsibility is to recognize these limits. Just as I suggested that we have a duty to fulfil the psychoanalytic promise to let the patient 'use' us to develop his own mind, we also have a duty to recognize when the 'use' becomes 'abuse' or it is simply not in the patient's best interests, all things considered.

When an analytic relationship breaks down, for whatever reasons, a deep sorrow must be borne by both parties—this is something that we don't discuss nearly enough within our discipline. It is an ethical labour to recognize the pain of an impasse that apparently cannot be resolved and to allow oneself to feel the sadness of this without retreating defensively into theoretical formulations that tidy up what is invariably the messy and nuanced reality of what went wrong. It is also an ethical labour to implement a plan of action that aims to stop an abusive or destructive (to the patient) cycle and protects the goodness of the work that has been done, where this is the case. We

must beware of how our narcissism or masochistic trends may interfere with the process of ending work with a patient and expose us to
the risk that we persevere in a repetitive cycle that is not helpful to
the patient. I have briefly digressed into these more exceptional cases
because they provide a good example of how the *ethical chóros* is a
place in our mind not only of conceptual ethical formulation and of
reflection on our errors or limitations. It is also the space where we
can register and work through the pain, guilt, and loss of a therapy
that has not had the opportunity to end in a planned fashion and/
or with a successful outcome. This work requires introspection and
confronts us with a very peculiar and challenging 'isolation', as I suggested in Chapter 1.

Kächele and Schachter (2014) also underline that we neglect
openly sharing information with new patients about possible treatment risks or negative outcomes. We expect a provider of medical
interventions to offer to the prospective patient an opportunity to
understand the risks or demands associated with the proposed procedure. Failure to provide such information would raise an ethical
concern. This expectation, they argue, is not prevalent in our field,
and we do not consistently discharge our duty to inform the patient
about what an analytic process entails. Clearly, it is much harder to
explain the vicissitudes of a psychoanalytic process and its risks than
it is to explain an appendectomy. That said, whereas in the past we
had relatively little information about psychotherapy outcomes, we
now have access to a body of work about the effectiveness of psychotherapy generally, and of psychoanalytic therapy specifically,
which can be shared in digestible form. Yet Kächele and Schachter
caution that,

> Based on our long-term clinical experience, psychotherapeutic prac-
> titioners seldom provide such information to prospective patients. We
> suspect it is because such information would have to include some
> statement about incomplete treatment and failure of treatment, and
> we believe that therapists continue to have difficulty acknowledging the
> presence of these common, significant negative events. (Kächele and
> Schachter, 2014: 248–249)

We would be better off as a profession if we could create spaces to reflect on treatment failures as an expected outcome, and importantly one from which we can learn and advance our discipline. It is of course much harder to define what is a 'good' and 'bad' outcome with respect to a psychoanalytic process than it is to evaluate whether an appendectomy has been successful or not. This, it itself, requires further thinking as a discipline and within each therapy. Nevertheless, without doubt, as I look back on my clinical work, the biggest learnings have resulted from experiences with patients where I got it wrong and/or where the patient did not leave feeling that the therapy had been of help.

Beyond our own individual resistances to recognizing failures, we cannot ignore the institutional resistances to acknowledging, reporting, and responding to treatment failures and transgressions. We have most data about sexual boundary violations and the institutional resistances to this have been well documented (Gabbard, 2015, 2016, 2017). The literature attests to a reticence to take concerns about colleagues' conduct seriously and to act promptly. This is especially so when the concerns relate to senior colleagues who may have been our teachers and inspirational figures in one's own development (Peltz and Gabbard, 2001). The obstacles to acting on a concern about a colleague lie at the foothills of transferential aspects of authority and power in analytic institutes and our own need to distance ourselves from awareness of our own vulnerability and errors. Slochower highlights how very difficult it can be to hold in mind contemporaneously the fallen idealized figure and their ongoing impressive capacities in some domains:

> Our need to deny what we know and to protect exalted mentors from scrutiny has led to a toxic collective silence; by and large, we have remained publically mute while engaging in plenty of private gossip. Anxiety about the destructive consequences of 'telling' further complicates our experience and can result in disavowal—a near total foreclosure of the reality of the breach along with our experience of it . . . . If we are to move beyond this impasse, we need to encompass the possibility that truly reprehensible professional behavior can

coexist with a capacity for good analytic work and intellectual brilliance. (2017: 195)

When a therapy is not helpful to a patient or where there has been a clear ethical breach, the ultimate responsibility rests with the individual therapist. However, we cannot ignore our collective responsibility to each other as colleagues and to the public to support and challenge each other when necessary (Burka et al., 2019; Gentile, 2018), and for creating spaces where we can critically reflect on our individual work and method.

Capacity, intentionality, and responsibility

'An ethic', as Lacan understood, '. . . consists in a judgment of our action' (1992: 311). Needless to say, our actions are informed by our *intentions* (conscious and unconscious) and are judged, first and foremost, by the intention that animates them (Atterton, 2007). We can consider actions as morally right or wrong, but we can also judge them morally good or bad. Both evaluations are logically independent of each other. An action can be right without being virtuous, but an action is virtuous only if performed in the right state of mind. For example, if a patient in our private practice asks for an additional session and we offer it, it makes a moral difference if we do this because we believe it to be in his best interests or if we do this because the request coincides with a time when we need additional income. The outcome is the same—we see the patient for the additional session—but the motivating state of mind is substantially different from an ethical standpoint.

Within ethics, the study of right and wrong action has been dominated by the opposition between teleology (consequentialism) and deontology. According to teleologists, the right-making qualities of actions are only their consequences. Deontologists instead insist that an action can be right or wrong *in itself*. Although I am not concerned here with applying virtue ethics to analytic work, I simply want to draw attention to how following ethical principles is necessary but not sufficient. As Sasha Nacht (2011)[5] put it, it is not what the therapist says or does that matter, but what she is. The willingness to be receptive to our mistakes, to openly scrutinize our intentionality towards the patient, and to take responsibility for what we do distinguishes the ethicality of the therapist.

We can approach the burden of responsibility that the therapist carries from another angle. In various ways, our intuitions suggest that we expect more of people with greater capacities in specific domains. A person who becomes more highly educated and trained often acquires new responsibilities that inform how her conduct in certain situations is then judged. For instance, a doctor who stands by in a group context and does not attend to a person who has a heart attack will likely be judged more severely (at least from a moral perspective) than the rest of the onlookers in the group who also did nothing but who lacked a medical training. This is precisely because the doctor possessed the capacity to potentially save that person, whereas the others did not. Of course, the person might die despite the doctor's intervention, but the ethical point is that the doctor acted based on her capacities and did her best. Turning to our profession, we might argue that a psychoanalytic therapist due to her training has more capacity to understand the human mind and identify the activation of different states of mind, such as a suicidal state, than, say, a teacher. This bears on how responsible we might deem the therapist to be if she failed to identify suicide risk in an adolescent patient where there are some clear warning signs, and who then attempts suicide, compared to the teacher of that same adolescent who also fails to identify the risk.

The philosopher Nicole Vincent (2013) argues that the responsibilities a person has are in part determined by what capacities she possesses (i.e. what she 'can' do) which, in turn, generate duties (i.e. what she 'ought' to do). In this sense, we might argue that greater capacity acquired through specialist psychoanalytic training affects

---

[5] 'Ce n'est pas tant ce que l'analyste dit ou fait qui compte, mais ce qu'il est' (Nacht, quoted in Denis, 2011: 81).

responsibility, hence blame. When a person has acquired a greater capacity in a specific domain, then we may hold her responsible for things for which previously (i.e. before her training) we would not have held her responsible. Vincent is not suggesting that we can 'read off' a person's responsibilities based on her capacities. It is far too simplistic to argue that 'can' always implies 'ought'. Rather, she suggests that in determining what responsibilities a person has, we should give due consideration to what capacities she possesses—that is our professional training, taken together with a range of other considerations, implies 'ought'. As therapists, we have a range of duties towards our patients. Because we have acquired highly specialized capacities in the application of the psychoanalytic method, we 'can' (theoretically) understand how things can go wrong in the analytic relationship. This 'can' suggests, at the very least, that we have more cause to question our ethics if we fall prey to the occupational risks that I will be shortly outlining. And if we do, then we are rightly held to be more responsible for these errors than someone who had no access to the understandings that we are privileged to acquire during our training. By emphasizing this, I do not wish to install at the heart of our work a persecutory analytic superego—no-one stands to benefit from that. However, it is incumbent on us to carefully reflect on the moral implications of our specialist training in terms of our responsibility towards our patients.

Occupational hazards

Every profession carries a unique set of occupational risks that potentially expose the 'professional' and their 'client' to harm. A scaffolder exposes himself to harm because he could fall during the job and the risk of this injury for him is consequently elevated. The scaffolder, in carrying out his duties, also exposes others to risk as the structure may collapse and injure his client or passers-by. Likewise, working at the delicately complex interface of internal and external reality, and across two minds who meet in the service of better understanding the mind of only one of the participants, presents risks to both therapist and patient and potential for harm. Some of the risks are inherent to the analytic setting in which the process unfolds (e.g. confidentiality; remote vs in person) and others result from the psychoanalytic method itself (e.g. the risk of regression and dependency).

Like all relationships, the analytic one exposes the patient and therapist to specifically *interpersonal* risks. It confronts both parties with the demands of separateness and difference as much as with the demands of dependency and intimacy. Forever precariously balanced on the tightrope of intimacy and its implications, we strive to take responsibility for the otherness of the other, as Levinas urges us to do (see Chapter 4). This responsibility is onerous and accounts for the hatred of the other that we need to manage in all our close relationships, along with love and concern for the other. As I suggested in Chapter 1, unless we can acknowledge how much we can love and hate our patients—sometimes in equal measure—we will surely make more ethical mistakes than if we can own the intense feelings that the psychoanalytic process may mobilize in both participants.

Our work exposes us to specific emotional demands. Donald Moss summarizes these:

> . . . the narcissistic vulnerability, the incurable sense of incompetence, the relentless inhibitions, the isolation, the brazen difficulty of being with oftentimes unpleasant patients, the diminished cultural stature of the profession, the sense of being a fraud, and other by-now-familiar features of what makes psychoanalytic work difficult. (2013: 122)

In a similar vein, Ackerman recognizes the importance of being mindful of what she calls the 'irreconcilable ideals' that we carry within us as therapists. She encourages us to engage with them rather than being driven by them:

> Each analyst must reconcile herself with these in order to arrive at a realistic approach to the ethical practice of psychoanalysis. With an appreciation of the confounding nature of our ethical aspirations, we can find a

way to engage these ideals, while also recognizing the inevitability of our tendency to fall short of them. (2020: 571)

Slochower too identifies how the analytic ideal sets up an unhealthy internal setting for the therapist that makes it more likely that breaches will occur:

Analytic misdemeanours may thus represent an unconscious rebellion against the ideal analytic position, whatever its shape, and an implicit, symbolic assertion of the analyst's subjecthood. These misdemeanours are virtually ubiquitous precisely because we find it so difficult to acknowledge openly and struggle with the clash between our very human selfishness and the still extraordinary demands of this 'impossible profession'. (2003: 468)

Finally, and in my view in one of the most challenging papers on this subject, Kravis (2013) names an important tension in his discussion of the therapist's 'feelings of imposture':

. . . analysts' feelings of imposture are amplified by their professionally instilled recognition of how far short they fall from the ideal of being paragons of mental health. They cannot but be all too keenly aware of the embarrassing ways in which their love affairs, marriages, divorces, relationships with their children, and dealings with their colleagues reflect their own character flaws. (Kravis, 2013: 98)

How true this is. As Lacan observed, 'The psychoanalytic act has but to falter slightly, and it is the analyst who becomes the analysand' (Lacan, quoted in Felman, 1982: 35). One day we are the one sitting behind the couch trying to help a patient take stock of why his marriage is falling apart. The next *we* may be the one in the solicitor's office signing our own divorce papers. One day we listen to an exasperated parent struggling with his rebellious adolescent and help them to set boundaries. The next *we* may be facing our own child's suspension from school. As we take up both positions—of being the therapist and the one who needs help—we need the space for the self-doubt ('I can't help anyone. I am the one who needs help') or for recognition of the resentment towards the patient for claiming mental space that we are short of as we face our own problems ('*You* think you've got problems . . .').

One (unethical) solution to the inevitable emotional demands that we must manage, is to set up with our patients what I referred to in Chapter 1 as *narcissistic pacts*. Therapeutic work presents us with opportunities to gratify our own needs, especially our need to be liked, to be needed, or to be a saviour, or to find in the patient a container for our pathology. Our self-esteem needs operate 'as ever-present forces in analysis as they do in life' (Jacobs, 2001: 667). I am always suspicious of any analytic relationship, especially when it extends over time, that shows no sign of any negative feelings from either party. It makes me wonder not only why it is not possible for the patient to see me as anything but good and helpful but also what it is that I may be failing to take up because I am invested in preserving a version of me as needed and loved by the patient. Losing sight of this opens us to the possibility of ethical breaches. For example, if we are turning to the patient for reassurance that we are special and needed, it may prove very hard to end a therapy that is not in the patient's best interests.

What follows, should in no way be considered an exhaustive list of the possible occupational hazards that we face, but its restricted focus aims to highlight broad categories that may lead to a range of ethical breaches, hence harm to the patient.

On hating our work

I love my work. I love accompanying people on a journey of self-discovery that I know from my own personal experience of psychoanalysis, can be nothing short of transformational.[6] I love doing work that, when it goes well, can make a tangible difference to people's

---

[6] In saying 'transformational' I don't mean imply that psychotherapy is a magical cure. There are many things that psychotherapy cannot change, not least our individual developmental history, our genetics, or the culture we are born into. But it can help us to manage our relationship to these givens in ways that are more enhancing of our well-being, all things considered,

lives. I am moved and inspired when I witness the development of a mind capable of overcoming traumatic past experiences and shedding defensive structures that once served the person well but now come with considerable collateral costs. I love learning more about the human mind and about myself through the challenges that each patient presents me with.

I also hate my work, sometimes. I love and I hate 'being used' by the patient as he forges his way through his own process, drawing me into his internal dramas, hating me, assigning different roles to me, sometimes roles that deeply jar, that I recognize I don't like because they push me to think about things that, for my own reasons, I don't want to think about. I hate the helplessness I can feel in the face of some of the experiences my patients report and my inability to help or to understand or the destructiveness this can mobilize in me and that I know I must accept if I am to reclaim the position of responsible agency that I have a duty to provide to my patients. I hate the loneliness of hearing so many painful stories that I cannot share because of confidentiality except, and all too briefly, in supervision.

I could go on, but I trust this suffices to make the point that helping people, and working psychoanalytically, precisely because we avail ourselves to 'being used' by the patient, is both a privilege and very hard work. As I suggested in Chapter 1, this means that there will be times when this leaves us hating the work and even hating a specific patient, in given moments, when we are in the grip of the demand placed on us.[7] Such feelings are commonplace in my experience of supervising colleagues and of reflecting on my own work, but we cannot underestimate the difficulty of sharing the hateful feelings because they can collide with a more idealized version of what a therapist should be like (e.g. always understanding, compassionate). It is as difficult to share these feelings as it is to share the attraction or

---

and it enhances our capacity to recover from future setbacks or losses with greater psychic flexibility.

[7] As I clarified in Chapter 1, when I refer to 'hating' the patient, I am referring to hating aspects of his behaviour and what he may be doing to us (e.g. humiliating us), and not the patient in any absolute sense.

love that we may feel towards a patient.[8] Of course, we need to ensure that we process the loving and hateful feelings without converting the very admission to these feelings into a virtuous state where, for example, the therapist who is admired is the one who can face her aggression and hatred towards the patient whilst the therapist who speaks to the loving feelings is seen to be avoiding 'what is really going on'. In practice, it takes courage to face *all* the feelings that our patients engage in us whether they are loving or hateful ones.

We often speak of the 'complex' patient. This can be a way of signalling that the patient has a range of needs, perhaps physical as well as psychological, that require input from different services, or it indicates the existence of psychiatric comorbidity and levels of risk. However, reference to complexity is also sometimes shorthand for a patient whom we experience as hard to engage or for the patient who is 'ungrateful' and appears to undermine our best efforts to help. Indeed, the patient's rejection of the therapist's efforts is a powerful trigger for enactments. We cannot ignore that some people are more difficult to help and to relate to than others. Being such a person's therapist is likely to be challenging. Just because we are the therapist, and even more so when we are trained to know about unconscious hatred and envy, we expect that we must take in, survive, and metabolize the patient's assault on us and not give voice with the patient to the destructive feelings this elicits in us. This is indeed what we must do. However, to do this, it is essential that we can also feel free (in ourselves) to experience feelings of resentment or imposition, for example, some of the time. Being truthful about what we feel is anchoring. When we are rooted in the reality of what we are feeling and reflect on it we can see more clearly the patient as separate from us and from who he has become in our internal world. Our relationship with the patient may well continue to be challenging, but we are less likely to feel frustrated or perhaps even persecuted by him.

As therapists we have a duty of psychoanalytic care that requires us to mentalize, for example, what may make it hard for the patient

---

[8] I am not defining here the type of attraction because it is not necessarily only of a sexual kind, but it is nevertheless always significant in terms of its impact on the analytic process.

to accept our help and to question why the patient may not be taking in what we are trying to communicate. This involves being open to the possibility that the patient may not be listening to us, not necessarily because he is attacking of our attempts to help (though sometimes this may well be true), but because he may find it hard to trust the truth and relevance of what he hears us saying. In such moments, turning the spotlight on ourselves can be illuminating. When the ethical impulse is mobilized, the frustration we previously felt towards the patient, gives way to consideration of how the situation might look from where the patient is standing. In this sense, we can see how our theories introduce specific risks: intersubjective and intrapsychic formulations respectively predispose us differently to how we listen. The more we lean into intrapsychic formulations in any given moment, the more we run the risk of potentially undermining the patient's reality sense by repeatedly reducing what he says to the activation of an internal dynamic rather than to something we may have also contributed to or are at the very least reacting to. Equally there are risks inherent to a purely intersubjective view, which may lose the focus on what the patient *is* initiating or 'doing' to his internal objects, and to us in the transference, and thus undermines a part of the psychoanalytic promise namely, to help the patient to understand his unconscious mind. I am not therefore arguing that there is a 'better' psychoanalytic stance, but rather that whatever stance we favour, it carries specific ethical tipping points.

Managing the challenges of asymmetry

Sexual boundary violations[9] are far more common than we would like to think. Studies from the United States indicate that the

---

[9] In the psychoanalytic context, Gentile draws attention to how the term '... *sexual boundary violation* displaces, if not disavows, both the action and the perpetrator. Certainly a boundary has been violated, and this should be taken up at the group level and understood to be a violation of the therapeutic relationship, the treatment, and the professional community, and institution as a whole . . . . But this term focuses on the violated boundary as if it were the primary victim, and only as an aside holds, or associatively alludes to, the fact that the *patient* was violated' (2018: 651).

incidence of erotic contact between patients and a group of mental health professionals pooled nationally from various disciplines (i.e. not exclusively psychoanalytic therapists) ranges from 7–12 per cent (Alpert and Steinberg, 2017; Borys and Pope, 1989; Jackson and Nuttall, 2001). As most of the studies typically rely on self-report, it is reasonable to speculate that this most likely underestimates the true prevalence. In the UK, it is hard to find much data—most of the research is from the US (Hook and Devereux, 2018).

In her 2011 paper, the psychoanalyst Muriel Dimen generously shared the painful experience with her male analyst when he kissed her at the end of a session. Although this 'slip of the tongue', as she put it, was never discussed between them, Dimen details how it took her years, literally, to name what had happened and come out into the public about her experience, though significantly she never named the analyst. One of the most moving aspects of her account is her description of how very difficult it can be to bring up these dynamics with the analyst and the pernicious impact this has on the patient:

> . . . So you don't notice, and you don't notice that you don't notice, and you don't bring it up, because you fear he will either disavow or acknowledge his role: if he's bad and denies it, then you're crazy, and if he's good and cops, then you have no right to be angry and your anger makes you bad and so it's your fault and, *voila*, you've no right to speak at all. And you don't tell anyone else because you don't want them to tell you to leave the analyst whom you need beyond reason. (Dimen, 2011: 72)

Such accounts are essential reading as they sensitize us to the corrosive impact of the silence that can entrap the patient and the painful bind it imposes on the patient. When the betrayal of trust takes place within a relationship regarded as trustworthy within society, this is graver ethically and in terms of the psychological consequences than other forms of betrayal. This is, in part, because it places the patient in the double bind of having to turn a blind eye to the betrayal to protect the needed relationship to the therapist on whom the patient depends for his care (Smith and Freyd, 2014). Jacobs (2001) suggests that for defensive reasons patients often suppress, deny, or rationalize their accurate perceptions of counter-transference elements (i.e. the therapist's needs and conflicts) and do not confront their therapists with it. He helpfully reminds us that even though perception is filtered through transferential and projective identificatory processes, the patient may yet accurately perceive aspects of our behaviour.

We must keep in view that unless we are prepared to openly discuss the erotic countertransference, during training and beyond, as an ever-present occupational hazard, we increase the risk of sexual transgressions. Avgi Saketopoulou specifically flags up the risks inherent to 'the de-sexualisation of the erotic countertransference' (2021: 117), which creates a dangerous slippery slope. However, as I have reiterated at various points, my primary focus in this book is not on the question of sexual boundary violations specifically and this is so for two reasons. First, there is now an ample and excellent literature that focuses on sexual boundary violations (see, for example, Levin, 2021). I don't have anything more to add to these very clear expositions of the problem we face except to outline how we might rethink training in ethics (see Chapter 8). Second, the focus on the more egregious ethical breaches conveniently diverts our attention away from the everyday ethical breaches that more subtly erode and corrupt practice, are easier to ignore or downplay in one's own mind, but are no less potentially damaging to patients.[10] It is essential to attend to how the very particular intimate nature of the analytic relationship carries significant risks that need not result in a sexual relationship with the patient but nevertheless create potential for harm to the patient.

The analytic relationship unfolds in the context of a paradox that defines the analytic setting. As Andrea Celenza (2010) helpfully frames it, it is a relationship that relies on the establishment of mutuality in the context of an asymmetry because the patient is the one

---

[10] For example, the published 2020 report by the British Association for Counselling and Psychotherapy on the investigated complaints reveals the very broad range of ethical complaints, not only sexual misconduct, available at: (https://www.bacp.co.uk/media/11019/bacp-ppc-annual-report-2020.pdf). Accessed June 2022.

seeking help such that his needs are the priority, not the therapist's. Celenza has articulated how the patient is promised understanding and non-judgmental acceptance whilst the therapist must dismiss her own needs during her work. This is difficult enough in any job, but even more so in the context of psychoanalytic work. This is because the experience and longing for intimacy that the patient brings invariably triggers that of the therapist, that is the analytic setting is stimulating, seductive, and frustrating for both parties. This deprivation sets the scene, as it were, for how the therapist may therefore be partially 'gratified and titillated' by the moments of attunement that the patient offers:

> It might be said that the frustration of asymmetry is counterbalanced by the seduction of mutuality and momentary attunements; 'we're in this together differently' mistakenly becoming 'we're in this together the same.' These vicarious identifications evoke and temporarily unsettle the analyst as he or she decenters and resonates with the analysand's experience. (Celenza, 2010: 64, original italics)

Our work is solitary much of the time: it is us and the patient, with short breaks in between, all day in the same room with minimal contact with people in the 'outside world'. Unless we work in an institutional setting, we will have limited or no access to being part of a team with colleagues that could provide interruptions and movement. On a busy day, we may not even have the chance to leave our room, keep up with the news, and learn about major national or international events as they unfold (Rokach, 2019). This exposes us to a kind of sensory and informational deprivation that can unmoor us. Because our work requires that we receive and immerse ourselves in another person's reality, it is also vital that we work in conditions that provide opportunities for grounding ourselves back in external reality and so regain our perspective and orientation in our reality.

Constant exposure to other people's pain, conflict, and sometimes acute disturbance, may also reactivate our own conflicts. As Welfel (2015) cautions, 'We repeatedly see the pain and destructiveness of people . . . . The cumulative effects of witnessing so much human suffering can wear down even the most competent professionals unless they are committed to self-care' (2015: 100). I am labouring over our typical 'working conditions' to remind us of the paradox we face every day when we go to work: despite the intense relational contact of psychotherapy, emotional isolation and a degree of sensory and informational deprivation are experienced by many therapists as a daily occurrence. The intimacy in psychotherapy is completely one-way, with the patient expected to share his world in detail while the therapist is not expected to react in kind; true mutuality is lacking. Focusing exclusively on our patients and their inner worlds may leave little room, if any, for attending to our needs and this may result in withdrawal from others who could otherwise provide support and perspective on our work.[11] Therein lie the seeds of burnout and of acting out.

Given the nature of our work, the scope for unconscious narcissistic pacts is therefore wide. This can result in what Levin (2021) terms 'narcissistic boundary violations', which involve 'an ongoing process of colonising the patient's mind, which may well take place in the absence of any sexual activity' (2021: 14). In our work, the possibility of 'colonisation' is all too real (Frosh and Baraitser, 2003). The asymmetry in the analytic relationship requires that the therapist manages the benign verticality of the relationship to ensure that it does not become a malignant verticality (see Chapter 1). This calls for ongoing self-monitoring throughout our career, including attending to our mental well-being. Ethical practice requires us to prioritize our own well-being so that we can avail our mind to the patient. Ignoring our state of mind and whatever stresses we may be experiencing exposes the patient to potential harm. The duty of self-knowledge thus extends to monitoring our own need for help and support and recognizing temporary or longer tern impediments to our fitness to practice (see also Section 3).

---

[11] For example, in their survey of 476 therapists, Pope and Tabachnick (1994) found that 20 per cent of respondents held a secret (over half of which identified as sexual in nature) which they would never to disclose to any other therapist.

Facing up to our needs and desires: Managing the boundaries around money, endings, and publication

Professional boundaries generally refer to the limits of a fiduciary relationship. That is, a relationship in which one person (a patient) entrusts his or her welfare to another (a therapist), who receives a fee for the delivery of a service (directly or indirectly). There are many situations that have the potential to exploit the dependency of the patient on the therapist and the inherent power differential in this relationship. An essential feature of the therapist's ethical labour is to grasp the responsibility we have for protecting the specific boundary between the patient and the therapist, without which the analytic space collapses.

A boundary demarcates two entities, or two parts of the same entity, which are then said to be in contact with each other. Boundaries are dependent for their existence on the entities they bind, that is the boundary exists by virtue of the two (or more) entities that require distinction from one another. The patient will have his own boundaries, but I am concerned here with the boundary *between* the patient and the therapist. The latter is an instance of a *fiat boundary*. Fiat boundaries are those induced through human demarcation, for example, in the geographic domain to separate adjoining countries. A patient and a therapist as a working couple have a boundary, but this boundary is not the property of either party—it comes into being *because* of the analytic relationship. Why does this matter? It matters because it alerts us to the way in which when we speak of a boundary violation, we are talking specifically about the violation of a boundary instantiated by the unique nature of the analytic relationship. A sexual relationship between patient and therapist, for example, represents therefore a *double* violation: it breaches the patient's bodily boundary, *and* it also breaches the boundary between patient and therapist.

Boundaries exist to facilitate the unfolding of the analytic process and to protect the patient from the therapist's self-interest and omniscience, that is our narcissism. We all vary in what we need and desire and the sense of entitlement that we have towards our needs and desires. When we think about boundary violations, as I referred to earlier, the literature provides many papers on sexual boundary violations and comparatively few on how other important boundaries may also be violated or manipulated thus harming the patient. Examples of the latter include when we publish a case without seeking consent or when we neglect reviewing whether a therapy is proving helpful and when it should end or how we manage fees. My experience with respect to these types of boundary situations is that they represent some of the most common triggers for when things go wrong. In the remainder of this section, I will focus on three needs in the therapist that can introduce ethical complexity: the need for money, the need to be needed, and the need for professional advancement. The first requires reflection on our conscious and unconscious relationship to money, which may also impact how we manage the length of a therapy. The second requires us to be able to know when to end a therapy rather than keep a patient in therapy because we regulate ourselves affectively through the patient's dependency on us or because of our financial dependency on the patient. The third entails careful consideration of confidentiality and of the use, in a publication, of what is the *shared* work of therapy.

Money

As a profession we remain deeply uncomfortable discussing money. The fees we charge when we work privately remain for many therapists a well-guarded secret that is seldom openly shared with colleagues. There are many reasons for this reticence, and I will not enter into discussing this. Suffice to say that our reluctance to discuss money can leave therapists feeling rather isolated around this issue, which accounts for why enactments around this boundary are commonplace.

One of the most concrete manifestations of the therapist's dependency on the patient is apparent when we consider the financial arrangements of private practice. The therapist needs the patient to attend regularly and to pay for his sessions. She needs this because she needs to earn a living in addition to exercising her choice of profession that pays dividends in other important ways too. If she works in a rented office, she has to pay her rent come what may; when patients cancel this has implications for her livelihood. For some therapists, money will be tight, and this can introduce complexities around cancellation policies. Holding patients accountable for payment of missed sessions underscores that 'missed sessions are not trivial events; they deeply involve both patient and therapist around commitment, finances, responsibility, self-interest, power, and reality' (Gans and Counselman, 1996: 43). However, the form that this takes varies and again introduces ethical challenges.

If we turn our attention to what remains the standard arrangement between many therapists and their patients, that is that the patient is charged for missed sessions unless the patient takes the same period of leave as the therapist, we do well to question how this arrangement can be ethically justified if a reasonable notice period is offered by the patient. Cancellation notice arrangements present a challenge to the therapist and her livelihood and clearly this is an issue, but it is hard to persuasively argue that the classical set-up is therefore primarily in the patient's best interests. Moreover, when we charge for a cancellation, especially where the patient gives us sufficient notice, it is incumbent on us to think through the status of the time that is freed up when a patient cancels and yet still pays the fee: what is an ethical use of this time? Should we be using it to think about the patient? What does it mean if during the time for which the patient is paying, we are working on something else?

Kurt Eissler (1974), in line with the classical Freudian position, argued that patients lease the therapy hour and pay whether they come or not as the 'rule of indenture'. He used the term 'gentlemen's agreement' for a less severe policy, one which absolves patients of payment when circumstances beyond their control occur or when adequate notice is given. In practice this is a complex position to take. Some therapists believe that not charging the patient for minor illnesses, for example, may burden the patient with guilt (Kreuger, 1986). At the other end of the spectrum, some suggest that the therapist should set a standard fee high enough to cover missed sessions due to the inevitable realities of life and consider that payment for missed sessions is the therapist's problem (e.g., Schonbar, 1986). Others still, such as Tulipan (1983), advocate that our fee and cancellation policies should be congruent with our personal style and attitude towards life. He did not charge for missed sessions. Instead, he decided how much money he needed to earn a year to maintain his lifestyle, took into consideration a number of hours per year that would most likely be missed, and developed a fee scale accordingly. This policy, according to Tulipan, helped him avoid the trouble that therapists are likely to encounter when they attempt to decide whether a cancellation is justified, and which inevitably sets up the therapist in the unethical position of omnipotence—the only one who can judge the validity of the patient's absence. Of course, when we know a patient well, we are better placed to assess the meaning of a cancellation, but it is also potentially difficult to operate a policy that we sometimes wave and sometimes not—'discretion' in these matters is ambiguous and runs the risk of playing into the power asymmetry that we must carefully manage.

We all have our own views about the meaning of money and the function it plays in the psychic economy of both patient and therapist. Considerations of justice may invite us to question whether we are systematically excluding certain populations from our practice through the level of our fee. However, deciding not to meet diverse needs, if we can direct the potential patient to an alternative appropriate source of help that is accessible to them, may be more ethical than accepting the patient into our practice and then resenting the low fee. Acting ethically in this respect is therefore not isomorphic with espousing predetermined values around money. Ethical practice does not require uniformity of practice and of policies. We each interpret how we manage boundaries such as fee setting or endings or publication. I don't believe that there is only one 'right' way to manage these. Moreover, what on the surface might appear to be more 'noble' positions, on further examination may reveal a more complicated picture. For example, a therapist who charges a modest fee is not inherently more ethical than the one who charges a high fee. The low-fee-charging therapist may seem on the surface to be more committed to social values and to put self-sacrifice before her own desires, but of course a low fee may also reflect unresolved issues around her self-worth and may paradoxically make it more likely that she is vulnerable, for example, to unconsciously ensnaring the patient into staying in therapy for longer than required because she needs the validation of being needed. The unconscious quid pro quo may be that the patient pays less but stays longer. Or the low-fee therapist may fear that if she charged high fees she would be viewed by colleagues as narcissistically entitled, overvaluing her own skills. The fear of colleagues' opprobrium may steer her in the direction of low fees, hence not primarily or only driven by her social values (Shapiro and Ginzberg, 2006). Morever, if a patient is very wealthy, we might question what it means to charge him a modest fee and what impact this could have on his view of the therapist and on the process.

The important ethical question therefore is not whether fees are low or high per se, but the reasons we have for where we set the fee and what policies we have in place if an existing patient is unable to continue paying or for making our services more accessible to patients who cannot afford to pay because this concerns matters of justice. We are responsible for having a clear, transparent system in place that communicates unambiguously what we can and cannot do and for monitoring that our decisions do not cause harm to a potential patient. The *transparency* of any policy is a precondition of its fairness (Rawls, 1973). In other words, those who are affected by a policy should be aware of it to ensure the individual can exercise his freedom in relation to it. Ethical practice requires us to be clear about our position, to measure it against the ethical principles we have reviewed, and to be transparent about it within ourselves and with the patient. These are essential considerations with respect to consent to treatment in the private sector.

Reviews and endings

The therapist's financial, and in some cases also emotional, dependency on the patient raises another thorny question, namely how we determine the appropriate length of a therapy or analysis. For the avoidance of doubt, I believe that each therapeutic dyad should decide what is right for that individual analytic journey. However, I am equally clear that this is a process that requires ongoing review of how the work is progressing and whether it's helping—however that is defined or contested as a legitimate aim of therapy. The patient may well decide that even if the therapy is no longer addressing the needs that originally brought him into therapy, that it has another important function and wants to continue for years. That strikes me as a very legitimate choice. By raising the question of 'reviews', I am therefore not arguing against long therapies or analyses. I am simply curious about the meaning of the resistance in much of our profession to building into our work regular reviews (e.g. in a long-term therapy, a yearly review seems reasonable). I am struck by how in long-term psychoanalytic work, the idea of a built-in review point would be mostly considered anathema and the therapist who does this is deemed to be straying away from the essence of psychoanalysis.

Of course, reviews are not unproblematic: some patients may relate to the review as a looming threat that the therapist may want to push him out and that the clock is ticking. This could be especially detrimental to patients who fear rejection or feel they have to perform and please the therapist in order to secure her approval. A review can introduce a temporality that works against the needs of a specific patient. We must not ignore these potential meanings. However, if the notion of a review is introduced at the outset of a therapy, in the context of seeking consent to the therapy, and is anticipated as a point of 'taking stock' to ensure that the patient feels that he is benefiting, then I am of the view that the benefits of reviews outweigh their risks. As and when the review takes place, we can name the anxiety this may give rise to (e.g. 'this is when you decide to get rid of me') and work through this with the patient.

We are ethically required to question any system of psychological care, of which psychoanalytic therapy is one, that does not routinely evaluate how the work is proceeding. Might it be the case that we are reluctant to introduce a review, not simply because this runs counter to the psychoanalytic canon of free association and a concern with not directing the patient, but because we are driven by a latent anxiety about being reviewed by the patient and/or discovering that the length of the therapy might be shortened if we introduce a review that allows the patient to realistically assess the value and progress of the work? A review can signal that the patient and/or therapist are continuing the therapy because separation cannot be faced. If the therapy is shorter, then the therapist loses work and must find more work. Moreover, we cannot ignore that working with the same patient over time may be less taxing in some ways since we will have established a degree of mutual understanding and a psychic map of the patient. Starting with a new patient requires a particular focus that makes renewed and different demands on the therapist. As someone who practices both brief and long-term psychoanalytic treatments, I recognize that brief therapy can be harder in some respects than an open-ended, intensive psychoanalytic therapy.

We may struggle to terminate a therapy for different reasons. Sometimes, the patient can become a source of love, care, concern, or stimulation and props up our self-esteem. He may serve the function of regulating our affects by providing us with a source of comfort that is otherwise missing from our life. Letting go of such a patient can be very hard, not least when the patient too derives gratification from taking up this role. As I mentioned earlier, narcissistic pacts are all too common and can interfere with our capacity to realistically assess when it is appropriate to end.

Finally, on the matter of endings, we cannot ignore the delicate and potentially painful question of knowing when we should stop seeing patients permanently or temporarily if our fitness to practice is somehow compromised. I recall many years ago now visiting my dermatologist to remove a mole that was worrying me. I had seen this dermatologist for decades. He was wonderful and highly regarded in his field. He continued to practice into his seventies and, on this occasion, as he took the scalpel in his hand, I noticed his hands tremble. I was both scared for myself ('How is this going to go?') and pained for him as I saw the man whose hands I had so trusted on so many other occasions, now vulnerable and fragile. He could still talk about cancerous growths with the same mental agility as he had done when he was younger, but on that day, it was clear to me that he should not really be practicing any surgical interventions, no matter how minor.

It sensitized me to the burden and guilt we may inadvertently place on our patients if they perceive a more sustained fragility in us because we are ill, or our memory is compromised.

In our work, we must face this truth: our capacity to be receptive to mental pain, our mental acuity, our memory, wax and wane throughout our lives reactive to temporary stresses and naturally, as we get older, we don't have some of the same capacities as when we started out. They simply decline, as I reluctantly observe in myself. Obviously, there are individual differences at play, and it would be inappropriate to generalize. However, the challenge we all face is recognizing that we will reach a point, for some sooner than for others, when it would be better for our patients if we stopped working as clinicians because what we offer may not be as good as what another colleague could offer. This is an ethical issue—one that is also narcissistically challenging. It is even more challenging in a field where the experience that comes with age is rightly prized but may obfuscate declining capacities to do the work of being a therapist specifically. Ethical practice requires of us as colleagues to help each other to see when we may have reached this point, no matter how painful. This is about taking care of each other in the analytic community whilst protecting patients from carrying the burden of anxiety and guilt of working, for example, with an increasingly fragile therapist. In his discussion about humility, Salman Akhtar discusses how the decision to continue working beyond a certain age may betray arrogance and raises ethical concerns. Importantly, he suggests that even though there is now greater awareness of these issues within the profession, this does not absolve us from reckoning with our narcissism:

> The denial of aging, increased potential for infirmity, and the proximity with one's own death [in such cases] is truly disturbing. Even under the rationale and rationalization of continuing good health, continuing to take on new analytic patients beyond a certain age carries not only a kernel of arrogance but also of compromised ethics; after all, one is knowingly exposing the new patient to the potential of a devastating loss. Fortunately, a trend is now evolving where matters of aging and

death are deemed topics for serious consideration. Many training institutes are setting age limits after which analysts may not take on new
cases in analysis. But this is externally imposed. What about the analyst's
own humility in limiting his or her professional career? (2018: 19)

It is not only age or illness that require us to consider our fitness to
practice. How we balance the composition of our work also deserves
consideration. Different pressures or changes in our private lives at
particular junctures may prompt the need to review the composition
or volume of the work that we do. Many years ago, I did a lot of court
assessments for refugees who had endured torture in their countries
of origin and were seeking asylum in the UK. During this phase of
my career, I became pregnant. At the time, I was given some very
helpful advice by a senior colleague who encouraged me to think
about whether it was a good idea to fill my mind with these horrific
narratives during pregnancy. I am grateful to her for raising this with
me and for her care. I heeded her advice and stopped undertaking
these assessments for a period. I also subsequently came to think that
it was not only in my best interests to stop this work, but that given
my role, it was not in my patients' best interests to continue. Stopping
this work was part of my responsibility towards them. Working with
trauma, and especially victims of torture, fills the mind with horrific
images that must be borne by the therapist. There is a limit to how
much mental anguish any of us can contain at any one time and this
limit is not static but reactive to what may be happening in our lives.
Knowing when we have reached our limit is essential if we want to do
the best by our patients and ensure the patient can work with a therapist who can avail her mind to him.

Such self-assessments can be difficult to initiate—I was fortunate
to be prompted by my colleague. In practice, there may be different
pressures that interfere with our capacity to take stock of whether
we are functioning optimally relative to what we have 'promised' to
offer our patients. For example, we may not be able to stop working
because we need to be the rescuer and our own vulnerability is projected into the patient or we may not have the option to stop working

because our livelihood depends on it. These are very difficult situations that require careful ethical analysis.

Publication of clinical material

Let us now turn to another psychoanalytic bugbear: confidentiality and publication. I dwell on this more than the other boundary issues because it involves revisiting the notion of consent, which is especially thorny in psychoanalysis.

The analytic relationship is bound by the requirement for confidentiality: no-one else but the patient and therapist can know about the work. Our relationship to notions of privacy and confidentiality can at times be very loose. Most patients correctly assume that our work needs to be discussed with a supervisor and that this is clinically necessary but few, I think, imagine that this may be done in a group setting, for example. Patients expect a near-exclusive commitment to privacy because they assume that their therapist would not discuss them outside of individual supervision or search online for them (see Section 4 for a discussion of Patient-Targeted Googling). Yet, regularly, patients are discussed in clinical seminar groups (e.g. during training) where the patient's identity is not adequately anonymized beyond withholding the name or occupation which, in isolation, does not offer much protection. Even when we ask participants in a seminar or at a conference to declare if they think they know the person who is being presented and to leave if this is the case, by that stage, if anyone does know the person, they also know the person is in therapy, so it is too late: confidentiality has been breached.

Typically, patient consent to publish clinical material is ethically required if there is any doubt about maintaining patient anonymity. If the case is unusual or if some details of the patient's history such as age or sex need to be given because they are material to the clinical or theoretical points the author wishes to make, and might therefore lead to identification of the patient, it would be necessary to obtain consent. Historically many therapists have published cases without seeking consent, using disguise and anonymization as a means of protecting confidentiality because this has been accepted practice, not because they are unethical therapists. This approach continues to be permitted under the International Psychoanalytic Association (2018) guidelines, which provide helpful and considered deliberations on this thorny ethical dilemma.[12] Nowadays we are more sensitized to the complexity of the issues at stake, which are not addressed by only disguising identifying features, not least because determining 'identifiability' is highly subjective. We might question whether the threshold for identifiability can reasonably rest with the author of a paper alone or also always requires the judgement of the patient.

Publication in our discipline is fundamentally an ethical issue for two reasons. First, because confidentiality is, as Jonathan Lear (2003) aptly puts it, 'constitutive of the process' (2003: 4)—if we breach this boundary through sharing clinical material beyond the context of supervision, we impact the foundational agreement necessary for the specific analytic process to unfold. It is of note that if the patient flags up at the outset of the therapy that he does not want us to use his clinical material in any way, we typically take this request to be binding. However, if the patient does not stipulate this, we appear to operate on the basis of an unarticulated 'opt-out' clause, that is we take the view that we can make the call about the appropriateness of publishing case material (albeit disguised) without necessarily seeking consent unless the patient explicitly 'opts out'.[13] This raises questions of fairness: many patients (typically more disadvantaged patients who are not acculturated with therapy) may not even think that their therapy might be used in this manner, and they could not therefore be expected to anticipate this possibility and state a preference. This

[12] Available at: https://www.ipa.world/IPA_DOCS/Report%20of%20the%20IPA%20Confidentiality%20Committee%20(English).pdf.

[13] Presuming consent as part of an opt-out system is not inherently unethical. The opt-out policy on organ donation is a case in point. If we look at the debates over that question, we find agreement from both sides of the debate that from a communitarian perspective, organ donation is a moral good and should be encouraged. However, and this is central to our concern with regards to publication, information about the opt-out process (e.g. through public information campaigns) is the key to ensuring the ethical validity of either approach.

leads on to the second reason why publication introduces an ethical challenge, namely that when we publish case material we are effectively 'using' the patient for a purpose that is not directly of benefit to the specific patient,[14] even if we could convincingly argue that it is of general benefit for the advancement of the discipline. The question is: is it ever ethical to 'use' the private disclosures of a patient without the patient's consent, even if the identity is disguised, having given the patient our assurances of full confidentiality?[15] And even if, for the sake of argument, it is established from a legal standpoint that disguising the material is considered sufficient protection and therefore defensible in law, this does not necessarily render 'ethical' the decision to not seek consent. Law and ethics sometimes overlap but they don't necessarily do so.

Introducing a request for consent to publish during an analytic process is an intervention in and of itself due to the impact this could have on the patient. A request by the therapist to publish, in the context of a relationship of dependency, inevitably also raises the question of the limits to informed consent. Once the analytic relationship is activated and subject to the dynamic and regressive pulls of the transference and countertransference, patient consent is an invariably complex question (e.g. is the patient agreeing in order to please us?). Gentile incisively points out that consent is more appropriately conceived of as always 'on the move', shifting along with the dynamics of the transference and countertransference.

> . . . Agency is complicated here because patients are to be experienced 'as if' they want what they say . . . . The patient's agency is to be analyzed rather than taken for granted . . . . Conceptualizing patients, or anyone for that matter, as incapable of giving consent can be disempowering, and . . . can seem patronizing, undermining notions of coherent,

[14] Helping an individual patient is the focus of presenting our work in supervision. Publishing a case is not routinely done in the service of the patient whose case we publish, even though I am sure that the process of writing up a case (without publishing) can be potentially helpful to the patient as it might help the therapist to clarify her own thoughts about the case.
[15] Of course, we may work under a restricted version of confidentiality, which would have been then specified at the outset of the therapy, say to accommodate intervening if there was a risk to life.

legible, and legitimate subjectivity. But we are not individual subjects. (2018: 653–654)

The indisputable complexity of what it means to give consent in the context of the transference is often used as an argument in favour of why it is meaningless to seek consent and hence the policy of 'thick disguise' of material suffices. The argument goes like this: the patient may not be aware at the time of giving consent to publication of the underlying unconscious motives for agreeing to this such that consenting may reflect other unconscious needs (e.g. wanting to please the therapist) that could not be deciphered within the time frame of a request for consent. Given this, seeking and receiving consent cannot deliver on its objective because consent is inherently unreliable. On the face of it, this is a legitimate concern. However, it is a dubious argument in favour of not seeking consent about publication.

Even though giving consent is complicated by the transference, we cannot ignore that if we subscribe to this view, then this would apply to any decision the patient makes or is invited to make during an analytic process, including for example, agreeing to the therapist's suggestion about increasing the frequency of his sessions or her fee or changing the session time when requested by the therapist. In such cases, we could similarly impute to the patient the potential, but as yet-unrecognized, unconscious motivation of wanting to please his therapist by agreeing to these recommendations or requests. If we held out on the presumption that the patient cannot meaningfully consent, we would reach a deadlock on all manner of things. Yet, when the decision concerns, say, agreeing to the therapist's suggestion of an increase in the frequency of sessions, we don't hear therapists routinely arguing that the patient cannot meaningfully consent to this. Rather, we tend to think that such an agreement is likely to be overdetermined, we explore the possible unconscious meanings and proceed on the assumption that most patients can nevertheless consent.

We cannot have it both ways. In other words, if we take a view of autonomy as all or nothing, then arguing that the patient cannot truly consent to publication due to the transference and the operation of the unconscious, is de facto tantamount to denying the possibility of consent to any decision pertaining to therapy. Our everyday practice suggests that we evidently do not adopt this view across the board, but we nevertheless use this argument to defend the right of the therapist to publish without seeking consent. Once we take this position, it then becomes all too easy to allow the entry of paternalism through the back door of ostensibly 'protecting' the patient. I suggest that we may be instead protecting our wish to publish without needing to enter the more demanding, messy interpersonal arena of seeking consent and working through the implications of this within the analytic relationship. This is indeed difficult—as I have discovered when I have sought consent—because it places us in the emotional fray of recognizing that we want something from the patient (for ourselves and/or for the profession) and that this need may potentially clash with the patient's needs, not least that his process is intruded upon by our request. Once we have asked the patient, we have introduced our agenda and hence our desire into the analytic space (Ackerman, 2018). This is not an argument against seeking consent—it's simply a measure of what we must contend with if we have good reasons for thinking that publication of a particular patient's experience will advance learning and benefit a greater number of patients.

When we decide against seeking permission so as not impinge on the analytic space, or because we consider that it could be detrimental to the patient to request consent, if the therapist still decides to publish disguising the material, the patient will not know this, but *we* know this. The act of writing, publishing, and presenting our work to others must have some impact on our mind and how we think about the patient. It is likely therefore to have some impact on the analytic relationship, not least when publication has not been discussed with the patient because it then becomes something of a secret. Either way, there is therefore a 'cost' to the patient. Moreover, if we strongly feel that to seek consent would adversely affect the patient, is this not an argument in favour of not publishing this particular piece of work so as to ensure that there is no possibility whatsoever that the patient would be affected by some of his experience entering the public domain, even if the risk is assessed to be remote?

We can make a strong (utilitarian)[16] argument in favour of sharing our work with others, not least the significant benefits to the public of a discipline open to scrutiny—one that can improve its therapeutic interventions through learning from its successes as well as treatment failures. Publication plays a key role in promoting this kind of culture (Tuckett, 2000) and advancing mental health care thereby potentially benefiting large numbers of patients. With all ethical matters, as we have seen, we need to balance competing duties and principles: the challenge lies in how we balance the value gained from publishing our work and benefiting future patients through the dissemination of knowledge that can improve psychoanalytic interventions *and* respecting the interests of the individual patient. The anticipated benefits of publishing our work support the argument in favour of publication but still leave open the question of the least damaging (to the patient) conditions for publication.

Given that there is a potentially adverse impact on the current patient whichever path we take (to seek consent or not) an important consideration that might help us to distinguish the least bad option, as it were, is to determine which option respects the patient's autonomy the most. When we focus on autonomy, it becomes clear that despite the intrusion into the analytic process, requesting permission to publish stands a better chance of respecting autonomy than doing so without seeking consent, notwithstanding the complexity of determining 'consent' in the context of the transference. Bypassing the patient's engagement in a process of thinking about what he feels regarding publication of material from his therapy is a form of paternalism and denies the patient all possibility of exercising autonomy over the use of his experience.

Publication of verbatim clinical material poses a further interesting question, that of ownership of the material. Given that detailed session material is ultimately co-constructed, is the work partly owned by the patient? Even if the disguise is watertight, when we report verbatim dialogue, we have nevertheless made use of the work of therapy, and specifically of words, images, or metaphors that

---

[16] Utilitarians argue that what matters is creating the most value across sentient beings.

are unique to the patient, without giving the patient the option of considering what he feels about this. We have ownership of how we understand the process and of how we write about it, but detailed dialogue cannot be considered to be solely the property of the therapist. I should specify that I am not concerned here with 'ownership' in any legal sense, but with our ethical position in relation to the shared nature of the material. The information the patient reveals as part of an analytic process remains, in a fundamental sense, their own. Anonymisation is effectively only a security measure. It does not change the ethical status of the 'data' as personal data. In this sense, anonymisation does not obviate the need for consent to publish case material.

The desire to share our ideas and to further our field are ambitions that in part at least reflect self-interest. They are legitimate ambitions and essential to ethical practice because sharing our work with others, improves our work. I am therefore not arguing that it is morally wrong to be driven by such desires or that we should not publish. I am suggesting that there are ways of pursuing these ambitions and our commitment to furthering knowledge that do not require us to unduly impinge on the patient's space or undermine his autonomy. For example, it is possible to construct a completely fictional case or to develop a fictional process dialogue that illustrates the clinical or theoretical point we wish to make—let's not forget that some of the richest learnings about the human mind come from fictional literature and that psychoanalytic authors regularly draw on fiction to illustrate clinical points, so we have established precedents that suggest there is merit in such illustrations. It is nevertheless true that fictional material cannot be taken to be 'evidence' in any scientific sense. That said, therapist verbatim reports of sessions are also subject to distortion, the vagaries of memory, and the post-hoc desires of what we wish we had said, so we might also question the status of this 'evidence'—short of a video or audio recording of a session, reported clinical material is always compromised. If we opt for fictional illustrative material, the challenge is that this is infinitely harder to construct than relaying a lived session, as we recall it. In other words, it is harder work for the author but not impossible.

I am strongly in favour of publishing, but if we do use an individual patient to share learnings in our profession, in my view, this can only ever be ethically justifiable with his consent.[17] In practice, it is very hard to identify an ideal time to introduce a request to publish that does not in some way impinge on the patient's space, which is why I have not published new detailed (i.e. verbatim) clinical material for several years now and have relied on composite cases. If I were to approach a patient in future for his consent, it would only be after a therapy has ended and some time has lapsed so as to not intrude into an ongoing process. However, even under such conditions careful thought would need to be given to how this could be experienced as intrusive by a particular patient.

As this brief discussion about the ethics of publication illustrates, we face considerable complexity when we approach any number of 'boundary' issues in our work, which is partly why it can be all too easy to cross a line even when we believe that we are acting in the patient's best interests. The best we can do is to think through carefully where we stand on the questions I have addressed in this section, challenge ourselves to unpack the assumptions that underpin the position we espouse, and ensure that our policies with respect to these boundary issues are clear and transparent. It is only through this kind of self-questioning and transparency that we can assess if there are inconsistencies in our thinking that merit being revisited.

The virtual slippery slope

Writing a book about ethics in 2022 requires consideration of the increasingly prevalent new setting for psychoanalytic therapy and psychoanalysis—the virtual setting. This introduces opportunities as well as risks. I will focus here only on the risks given my concern with occupational hazards. The constantly shifting horizon of emerging

---

[17] I will not enter into a discussion about 'exceptions' as that is too detailed for our purposes in this chapter but suffice to say that there are special considerations, for example, work with children.

information technologies requires us to be alert to new forms of en-actment and breaches. The complexity and evolving nature of the moral dilemmas presented by such technologies provide a good illustration of why our ethics cannot be enshrined in a fixed code but need to be responsive to the changing world around us. This exposes the insufficiency of universal moral principles in the absence of the contextual sensitivity to, and ability to read the moral significance of, the changing external contexts in which we live and work. The specifically ethical issues raised by the virtual setting should by now be fully integrated into our training curricula, but this is not yet the case in many trainings.

We cannot escape the fact that digital technology tethers humans and machines like never before. It is not simply that new media have created a new way of being-in-the-world, but they have also changed how we work. The in-person and the virtual setting may be equally effective for some patients, and perhaps the virtual setting is more effective for others, but they cannot be considered functionally equivalent and for some patients it is, in my view, contraindicated. Moreover, working in digital times, and especially post the Covid-19 pandemic that normalized remote therapy, introduces new risks. This is primarily because the altered contingencies afforded by virtual space impact in highly specific ways on our capacity for self-governance.

Virtual space operates like a cocoon, with none of the usual referents that might give pause for thought or impose limits on what it is possible to do thus making it more likely that we behave in unethical ways. The virtual setting more readily corrupts superego functioning (Wood, 2011) and moral integrity (Van den Hoven and Cockin, 2018). Suler (2004) has written about the 'online disinhibition effect' that is characterized by the following: dissociative anonymity (what I do cannot be traced back to me); invisibility (no-one can see what I look like); asynchronicity (my actions do not occur in real time); solipsistic introjection (I can't see the other(s) so I have to guess who they are and their intent); dissociative imagination (these are not real people); minimization of authority (I can act freely). Several of these features are not relevant to remote therapy via Zoom, for example, because it is a visual medium where both participants are known to each other. However, the last two features, 'dissociative imagination' and 'minimization of authority', pose risks precisely because virtual communication does not require our embodied presence in the same space as that of the patient: as the body becomes unmoored, it can precipitate action rather than reflection and this is a breeding ground for ethical breaches (Lemma, 2017). Working remotely may shift the therapist's representation of the patient to being that of a 'virtual other' and make a range of ethical breaches more likely.

A good illustration of the new risks introduced by the Internet is the problem of 'Patient-Targeted Googling' (PTG). The Internet has changed psychotherapy significantly since Freud's time and not only with respect to the physical setting. For example, the therapist's anonymity can no longer be guaranteed. Patients routinely look us up online before they meet us and sometimes during a therapy. For therapists, it is equally easy to find out a lot of information about patients. PTG refers to a healthcare professional using the Internet to discover information about a patient. That this happens far more than is admitted to within our profession, is not in question (Kolmes and Taube, 2014; Pirelli et al., 2016). The prevalence of PTG has been documented among medical professionals (e.g. Jent et al., 2011; Omaggio et al., 2018) and psychotherapists (e.g. Eichenberg and Herzberg, 2016; De Araujo and Kowacs, 2019), although the implications of PTG are likely to vary depending on professional group. Kolmes and Taube (2014) found that almost three-quarters of a sample of mental health professionals who had conducted PTG did not explore this in supervision. Feelings of shame, or fear of disciplinary action are likely to discourage disclosure, and hence constructive reflection on this dynamic. There are also generational factors at play: PTG is more likely in therapists who have trained after 1980—the digital native generation (Vodanovich et al., 2010). Membership in the digital native demographic is associated with a new and different social etiquette in which the collection of another person's data is viewed as socially acceptable (Ellison et al., 2010; Lyndon et al., 2011) and PTG may not even register as a problem in the therapist's mind.

PTG includes not only use of Google as a search engine but also encompasses all Internet-based searches including Facebook and other social media (Clinton et al., 2010). Although Internet postings are in the public domain, viewing information that a patient has not specifically shared in therapy requires careful ethical consideration. Some of our searches may start with a clear therapeutic goal, such as gaining an understanding of an adolescent patient's online avatar, but this initial rationalization may escalate to reveal other more ethically troubling motivations which, pre-Internet, would have been inhibited. For example, pre-Internet we might have been curious about where the patient lives, or what his partner looks like, but if such curiosity had been aroused, most likely we would have been deterred from giving into it, by the concrete steps we would have needed to take: to physically leave our house and drive to look at our patient's house or by the need to ask the patient for a photo of his partner. These would be such concrete actions that most of us would likely refrain from acting on these. However, the privacy of the internet, and the ease with which we can intrude other's lives without their explicit consent, and without anyone needing to ever know about it, creates a new risk of harm. The ethical problem is not only that we have invaded the patient's privacy. It also concerns the impact on the analytic process and outcome of what we discover because it exists in our minds: it becomes a guilty secret, something known but not shared and this is corrosive to the analytic relationship in much the same way if we publish material from a therapy without seeking the patient's consent.

A separate but related risk of remote therapy, and the use of media such as texts and emails in the context of an analytic process, is that they are seductively informal such that the therapist can all too easily find herself on the slippery slope of virtual relating. The so-called slippage arises partly because Zoom or texting, for instance, engender a relaxation of the boundaries of the setting. Indeed, sometimes the very notion of 'setting' becomes increasingly loose. For example, it is not uncommon for patients to use Zoom via their cell phones and carry out their session in the most unlikely of places (e.g. a park, a taxi). Likewise for therapists who may start to offer

Zoom sessions from locations other than their own consulting room setting.

Because the setting is potentially felt to be more 'relaxed', and in some respects more gratifying, it is easier to slip into enactments when working through the virtual medium. The absence of the two bodies in a shared physical space also plays an important part. Some argue that a virtual relationship protects the patient who may be anxious about sexual or aggressive transgressions by the other. Paradoxically, however, it is precisely because of the physical proscription imposed by the fact of mediation that problems arise. When the actual bodies are not directly implicated, the relationship that unfolds in a virtual space can more readily become seductive: the fact that 'nothing can happen really' (i.e. 'I am in love with my therapist but we can never consummate the relationship because we are not in the same room') seduces both patient and therapist away from reflecting on what *is* nevertheless happening between them at the level of fantasy. The frame of a physically co-present context is vital, I am suggesting, for protecting patient and therapist from the slippery slope of virtual relating. When both bodies share the same space, the somatic countertransference can be more easily noted and relied upon with greater confidence, and this can minimize enactments.

Indeed, it could be argued that erotic excitement—a normal and expectable response in an analytic dyad—can function as a cue to take note of what is happening in our body and reflect on its meaning in the context of the work with the patient. When such excitement occurs through mediation, and the whole experience can be written off as 'virtual' and hence not real, the risk of transgression can be minimized in our mind, and we may consequently be less attuned to it. The danger is that the virtual meeting encourages a 'pretend' state of mind in both participants where psychic reality is decoupled from external reality. And yet even if the therapist and patient do not physically act on each other's bodies, they can still act powerfully on each other's minds with detrimental consequences for the patient if the therapist does not remain watchful of the transference-countertransference. Co-presence stands a better chance of helping the therapist to identify and analyse physical sensations that protect against acting out in response to the emergence of loving and erotic longings.

The pandemic has obfuscated the clinical and ethical considerations pertinent to remote work because it left all of us, for varying lengths of time, and depending on which country we worked in, with no alternative. However, what is 'better than nothing' in some circumstances is not necessarily better in any absolute sense. Nowadays, and consequent to the pandemic, hybrid ways of working have become more normalized. Some therapists have welcomed this as it offers them, for example, more flexibility to work away from the location of the consulting room by offering remote sessions. We cannot categorically claim that hybrid ways of working are always a 'bad' thing for all patients. However, it's clear that the hybrid setting is not necessarily in all patients' best interests. In fact, I suggest that any such offer initiated by the therapist or requested by the patient deserves exploration. If hybrid working is suggested by the therapist to meet her needs (such as to be able to take longer breaks or pick up children from school), this would be a clear example of a therapist's needs taking centre stage. In such instances, where a need for an altered setting emerges, it is important to examine whose interests are being met.

Remote working may at times be necessary in order to enable work to continue that would otherwise not be possible. Through the experience of the pandemic, we have learnt more about how we can work most effectively through this medium and the opportunities this offers are as important as the risks I am focusing on here. However, it is hard to see how we could convincingly argue that remote work is a better or unproblematically equivalent way of working when in-person work poses no threat and is geographically feasible. There are some interesting exceptions to this last statement such as the needs of patients with avoidant personality traits or those who struggle with marked shame about the body, and for whom the in-person setting can prove so challenging that remote work can be a safe first, 'better' step and provides a facilitative bridge to in-person therapy, eventually. So, there are potentially sound clinical and ethical justifications for remote work in specific cases, but I suspect that we would be serving selfish interests, or striving to cut costs if in public services, if we continued to offer remote work routinely without questioning such an offer and ensure we have good reasons for doing so (i.e. it is in the patient's best interests).

These are not arguments against remote therapy but merely a reminder that it is a complex arrangement that is not indicated for all patients. The experience of enforced remote working during the pandemic has made it all the clearer to me that whilst some patients do just as well through this medium, some are significantly disadvantaged by it, either because their difficulties cannot be addressed well-enough through this medium (especially where the patient's embodied experience is a central feature of the work) or because the therapist cannot respond as well to their needs remotely due to her own personal aptitudes and/or preferences or a combination of both.

We do well to remember the importance of abstinence in our work, as Freud (1919) emphasized. He proposed that once the therapist becomes an important object to the patient, that is, once she becomes invested as the target of transference wishes, the therapist should leave these wishes ungratified and instead analyse the defences that develop. Clinical experience repeatedly demonstrates that affect soon emerges in response to the experience of frustration along with the accompanying phantasies that are elicited and the defences to manage this. This allows the therapist to help the patient examine his conflicts. In other words, abstinence gives rise to a state of deprivation crucial to treatment. However, we now live and work in a world where a 'state of deprivation' has little currency, if any at all: desiring, waiting, and frustrations are encumbrances rather than states of mind that bear their fruit when tolerated (Lemma, 2017). This shapes the expectation patients have of therapy and that we can sometimes also share, namely that therapy should be provided no matter what or where, when needed. The therapist too needs to renounce gratifications if she is looking for these to be met by the patient and how the work unfolds. Like anonymity, the optimal state of deprivation that Freud regarded as crucial to treatment is undermined in our current practice in the digital age. Remote therapy can be experienced as deeply gratifying. It can feed into fantasies of greater intimacy and of ease of access to the therapist. These may be left unexplored because the use of the virtual medium can be all too easily rationalized in a world where mediation is the norm.

In this chapter, I have emphasized that psychoanalytic therapy takes place within the highly seductive context of therapeutic asymmetry and increasingly within a virtual setting. This means that the therapist is inevitably exposed to occupational hazards. I have also underlined that we should not hide behind a focus on egregious violations and our moral conjectures about how such scenarios can arise, because this more readily results in us ignoring our 'everyday delinquencies'.

The *ethical chóros* supports our ability to think through clinical dilemmas or errors without giving way to denial or splitting that locates the problem elsewhere. This is an individual process that is aided by our own therapy and supervision but it also requires sustained institutional effort to prioritize thinking about ethics during training and beyond it—themes we will return to in Chapter 8. I imagine that no therapist would take issue, in principle, with the basic ethical tenet explored in this chapter, namely that when things go wrong, the therapist should take responsibility. I imagine, however, that there will be differences in how therapists understand the nature of the 'wrongness' and how they believe this is best approached with a patient. We turn to the latter in Chapter 6 and focus on the function(s) of apologizing.

6

Apologies Matter

Never ruin an apology with an excuse.

—(Benjamin Franklin)

The public's expectation is that therapists—like any other person involved in the helping professions—will always behave ethically. When there is a breakdown in this expectation, the breach of trust has grave consequences not just for the patient but also for the standing of the profession. The expectation of the highest standards of ethical behaviour extends to us all. However, as we saw in Chapter 5, we are all liable to getting it wrong and ethical breaches do occur. *How* we respond in these situations matters. It is incumbent on us to approach our mistakes with humility[1] and recognize the moral and clinical value of apologizing when things go wrong. Ideally, we offer an apology because it is merited and it is in the patient's best interests.

Regrettably, the possibility of legal action has perverted the ethical value of an apology in and of itself. In an external climate that has become increasingly litigious, there may be pressure to not apologize—an expression of contrition for an error—for fear that it may be seen to be an admission of liability. I do not engage with this question here because it distracts us from an examination of the psychological and ethical merits of an apology. The latter is the focus of this chapter, which is best read as a discussion of the architecture of an

---

[1] Salman Akhtar (2018) draws attention to the striking paucity of psychoanalytic literature about 'humility' given how central we would think this would be to our analytic stance: 'This lack of attention to humility is puzzling' (2018: 1).

apology and its interpersonal function. In discussing the function of an apology in the context of the analytic relationship, I want to draw attention to some of its constituent elements so that it does not become an 'inflated form of moral currency' (Smith, 2008: 4).

The Duty of Candour (DOC)

Following the scandal in England at Mid-Staffordshire NHS Foundation Trust between 2005 and 2009, where there was found to be a gross failure to review and respond to patient safety incidents, the Francis Inquiry (2013) recommended that all health care providers have not only a professional but also a statutory Duty of Candour (DOC) with their service users. In the medical context this applies when a patient safety incident has occurred that has resulted in death, severe harm, moderate harm, or prolonged psychological harm.

The DOC first came into effect in England in November 2014. The new legislation[2] introduced a statutory DOC for health care providers to ensure a legal obligation to be open and truthful with patients when things go wrong with their care. The medical community has long regarded the disclosure of harmful and 'non-harmful' error as a fundamental tenet of ethical practice and a necessity for patient care. Recognition of error is a prerequisite for an apology, which is a morally salient component of the process of amending any therapeutic error or breach. The DOC essentially refers to the process of talking openly and honestly with a service user and their family when harm has occurred owing to an act or omission by a health care provider. Moreover, providers are expected to engage the DOC process regardless of whether the service user has complained and even where he is unaware that a patient-safety incident involving him has occurred. The spirit of the DOC is primarily about changing institutional culture and giving prominence to the necessity of openness

---

[2] Health and Social Care Act 2008 (Regulated Activities), Regulations 2014, Regulation 20.

and honesty when things go wrong. In short, it is about avoiding cover ups.

In 2021 the British Psychoanalytic Council (BPC)—the UK registering body for psychoanalytic practitioners—ushered in a DOC to complement the BPC's code of ethics. This new duty, as it is articulated by the BPC, specifies that the therapist must be 'candid' with patients when something goes wrong with their treatment or care and causes, or has the potential to cause, harm or distress. The BPC outlines that given the specific nature of the analytic relationship this harm may be caused, for example, by misunderstandings or breaches of confidentiality. It goes on to clarify that:

> Being candid with a patient should not be misunderstood as admitting liability or wrongdoing nor should it be confused with complaint handling. The Duty of Candour applies irrespective of whether a complaint or concern has been raised by a patient and any action taken should always be in the best interests of the patient.

In other words, the guidance suggests that while apologizing is always the right thing to do, saying sorry does not imply liability or fault. The revised code of ethics further details that the therapist must:

- Tell the patient when something has gone wrong.
- Apologize to the patient.
- Offer an appropriate remedy or support to put matters right (if possible).
- Explain fully the short- and long-term effects of what has happened.[3]

The DOC thus enshrines in the code of ethics a new demand for the therapist. This is a positive development. However, the DOC ushers in a requirement that some therapists may find confusing (the BPC, after all, is only giving an outline guidance and cannot dwell on

---

[3] Available at: https://www.bpc.org.uk/professionals/registrants/duty-of-candour.

specifics) and that some will also find to be at odds with how they have traditionally approached, say, a misunderstanding in the context of the analytical dyad.

The ethics of an apology

Central to the DOC is the necessity for the therapist to take responsibility and to apologize. The assumption of responsibility begins not with interpretation but with an honest acknowledgment that something has gone wrong and that we are sorry. Apologizing recognizes that something could have gone *better*. It is the first stage towards learning from the 'incident' and preventing it from reoccurring. It allows for steps to be taken to mend the relationship between the patient and the therapist after an incident. In Chapter 1, I defined the responsible therapist as the one who makes a unique psychoanalytic promise to the patient: I will allow you to 'use' me, within the clearly defined context of the analytic setting, to serve your best interests in developing a mind of your own. When we break this promise, harm can occur, and this calls not only for acknowledgement but also for apology.[4]

The evolution of the concept of an apology reveals two trends that can still be traced today in the ambivalence many of us betray when it comes to apologizing for a mistake. On the one hand, we associate apologizing with confession and remorse. On the other hand, the apology may be no more than a concealed form of defence or rhetorical strategy. Plato's *Apology* is often taken as the starting point of discussions on the apology. *The Apology* is an account of the speech Socrates makes at the trial in which he is charged with his failure to recognize the gods believed in by the state, instead inventing

---

[4] Formal complaints processes make it clear that therapists are sometimes accused by their patients of something that they have not done, even if the patient experiences an all too painfully 'real' wrongdoing in his internal world and attributes it to the therapist. I could not access any published material on the respective percentages but I would expect false accusations to be in the minority. Complaints that are not upheld are not necessarily an indication that the patient fabricated their account.

new deities and thus allegedly corrupting the youth of Athens. Paradoxically, Socrates is anything but apologetic in his response as the term has come to be understood in contemporary culture. Instead, he provides an *apologia* as was customary in the classical Greek legal system: a rebuttal to the prosecution's accusations, which is a defence of his position. The modern use of apology as an admission of wrongdoing rather than a defence seems to have gained momentum around the sixteenth century, when it became linked to the experience of 'regret' (Smith, 2008).

In bioethics, the consensus is that after initially disclosing the raw facts of an error, a clinician should deliver a cogent apology to honour the moral worth and dignity of the patient who was wronged. Traditionally, such an apology requires acknowledgement of inappropriate action (often contained in the 'disclosure'), recognition of responsibility, expression of regret, and intention to avoid a repetition in the future. In this sense, an apology is a *constitutive*, or performative, action. Unlike constative speech (e.g. saying 'I am talking' while telling a story), apologizing is constitutive, that is the very expression 'I am sorry' is the act itself. In practice this means that it is not enough for a therapist who erred to think to herself or with her supervisor, 'I did something wrong. I feel bad. I won't let that happen again'. These feelings must be externalized with the patient in a speech act to reflect a true apology.

Another way to think about an apology is to view it, as Rapport suggests, as a kind of claim to knowledge and/or a claim to responsibility: 'as a claim to knowledge, an apology says that I know of a situation that I wish had not occurred; or else I know of a situation which I know you would wish had not occurred' (2009: 349).

As a claim to responsibility, at its most sincere, an apology clearly situates the locus of responsibility for the problem with one party, validates that there is a relationship that matters and is worth repairing, and thus communicates the value of this relationship. However, it is precisely around the claim to responsibility that we can discern slippage whereby the apology becomes an excuse. There are two types of excuses: in one we accept responsibility but deny that what we did was bad, or we dilute its impact on the patient, and in the other we admit that what we did had an impact but don't accept full, or even any, responsibility. My own post hoc self-reflection about the kinds of apologies I have sometimes made in my private life, and to my patients, alerts me to a bias that I imagine is not restricted to me: because a true apology requires so much of the person apologizing, apologies may contain degrees of denial, deflection, or justification of actions to restore our own perception of damaged character. From a semantic standpoint, regret, or concern— 'I'm sorry this happened'—is not at all the same thing as a fully fledged apology. Shame about our actions can all too often lead to expressions of self-justification. By contrast, guilt drives the mature apology. This denotes functioning in a depressive position, which motivates the desire to repair.

Between an expression of sympathy or regret and an acceptance of blame, there is potential for fudging the question of responsibility. Our choice of language can betray this. For example, if a therapist recognizes that she has repeatedly been emotionally absent in sessions after the patient draws her attention to this and says to the patient "I am sorry *if* you have experienced me as not available to you over the past few sessions", such a statement conveys a very different meaning to an admission that, 'You are right. I have been distracted recently and I am sorry that this has left you feeling abandoned when you need my help'. Although this distinction seems rather obvious, the expression of sympathy is often the hallmark of the 'safe apology' guidance, such as the one embedded in the BPC's DOC. This can send a mixed message to the patient. Although we are increasingly operating in a legal context where admission of wrongdoing may make us legally liable, my point here is not about the law but about ethics. An apology that is no more than an expression of sympathy for the patient's subjective experience rather than an acknowledgment of an action or omission by the therapist towards the patient loses its ethical muscle. Words matter because words are also actions and communicate our values. An excellent example of an unambiguous apology is the fulsome public apology offered in 2022 by the Finnish Psychoanalytic Society for the views expressed historically by Finnish psychoanalysts about homosexuality and gender diversity, which they now recognize have caused harm to patients in treatment. The statement they issued was unambiguous, non-defensive, and assumed full responsibility.[5]

There are scenarios where the expression of regret is appropriate because we are not morally responsible for the alleged wrongdoing even though something 'bad' has happened—this is what is typically referred to as 'agent regret'. In such instances, we may be responsible but not morally blameworthy. The philosopher Bernard Williams (1981) discussed 'agent regret' in his broader account of moral luck. In Williams's classic example, a truck driver, 'through no fault of his own' (1981: 28), runs over a child; the driver is causally responsible for the fatal accident, even though he is not morally blameworthy. Williams suggests that the driver experiences agent regret because the effect (or outcome) of his action—unintended harm—conflicts with the kind of impact he wants to have on the world (i.e. to not be someone implicated in the death of child).

By way of an example relevant to our work, imagine that we are mugged on the way to our private consulting room carrying our patient's notes (which we keep at home for safe keeping because we are in private practice, and we carry these to work each day). The notes are stolen along with everything else. In such a scenario, we would likely experience regret that the patient is exposed to a breach of his confidentiality, but we would not be considered morally blameworthy or even in breach of the code of ethics (notes cannot be stored in a part-time rented room that is shared with several colleagues, and we are not responsible for being mugged). Yet, we must manage being a therapist who has not been able to protect her patient's confidentiality, even though we are not morally responsible for the loss of the notes.

So far, I have focused on what constitutes an apology but not on why apologies are intrapsychically and interpersonally important. An apology is important because regret has a valuable *communicative* function. When something has gone wrong, an apology restores

---

[5] https://psykoanalyysi.com/wp/julkinen-anteeksipyynto/. Accessed July 2022.

epistemic relationships, of which the analytic relationship is one. Regret functions to close the epistemic gap between ourselves and others. As human beings, as I have suggested throughout, we only have indirect and fallible access to our own and each other's minds. An explicit expression of regret, as with other emotions, clarifies both to ourselves and to others where we stand with respect to the choices and the decisions we make, the actions we perform, and the outcomes we cause. When the therapist non-defensively acknowledges a mistake, and this practice is transparent, the patient is more likely to regard what the therapist says as legitimate, to learn from this experience, and generalize the learning to his life, despite the experience of a breach.

Jeffrey Helmreich's (2015) philosophical account of regret and of the apology deserves reading. He draws a distinction between two kinds of harm. In the prototypical case, a 'wrong' action causes a particular harm to the victim. For example, if I share a consulting room with you and I take a book that belongs to you without asking, perhaps because I assume you won't mind my doing so (and I need it urgently for a paper I am working on), but I then lose the book, one harm is the loss of your book. However, Helmreich suggests that in this type of scenario, another kind of wrongdoing has been perpetrated, which expresses something disrespectful or otherwise harmful to you, apart from the harm involved in taking your book in the first place. This further effect is what Helmreich calls an 'expressive harm', that is the action (taking the book without asking) expresses the implicit attitude, 'I can treat your possessions as my own' or more generally the attitude, 'it is acceptable to mistreat and/ or harm you'. Given this distinction, Helmreich's point is that an apology can counteract expressive harm, and it is this that allows for moral repair (i.e. through addressing wrongdoing) if the apology is accepted. This results because the apology acknowledges not only what I have taken from you (the book) but also reveals to you my recognition of your right not to have been mistreated by me. One implication of this analysis is that restitution is then not sufficient for moral repair: if I take your book without asking and then lose it, replacing it could address *that* harm, but replacing the book does not address the expressive harm. It does not acknowledge the disrespect in so far as I behaved as if your book is for me to take and to use as I like. When something goes wrong in the analytic relationship, the apology therefore needs to address the expressive harm because this is instrumental to the possibility for repair of the 'relational gap' that has been exposed by the breach (see Chapter 5).

An apology cannot correct all or even most of the damage wrought by a wrongdoing. Words won't undo the harm caused by a therapist, for example, who sexually violates a patient. If this is true and yet we consider that apologies perform moral repair, what aspect of the wrong can an apology change? Besides the question of truthfulness, which is the kind of authenticity that is carried by the therapist's apology, there is also the question of the value of an apology. You will recall that Helmreich suggests that a wrongdoing involves a certain mistreatment of the victim, over and above what else it inflicts on her, that is acting towards her as though it is acceptable to wrong her as we did. An unambiguous apology thus entails a commitment to a *shared value*, which speaks not only to the prospect of a future free from harms caused by breaches of the shared principle but also to a relationship that restores a sense of trust in a just and fair world. The worth of the apology by a therapist lies precisely in the restoration of epistemic trust, which is of value to the patient because the therapy is redundant without it.

We might think of an apology as a form of interpersonal, temporal punctuation. The relationship between apologizing and temporality is indeed worth noting. The apology functions to mark a new moment in the present that is linked to the past but that looks towards the future rather than the focus being on rewriting the past and an orientation towards the past. The act of apologizing signals to the patient that he matters enough for the therapist to seek to repair the pre-existing relationship with him. The apology effectively states, 'I did wrong, and I apologize, which will not make up for the wrong, but I acknowledge the wrong done'. Thus, the apology accomplishes what the French philosopher and sociologist, Jean-François Lyotard, referred to as the offering of the statement, 'It happened' (1983: 106). This is an important form of 'witnessing'.

Apologies are also psychologically important for the person who has been harmed because of the 'emotional re-balancing' (Vines, 2007) delivered by an apology. An apology repositions the affected persons. It humbles the therapist and builds the patient's self-esteem and reality testing through the process of recognition (Akhtar, 2002). This is the aspect of the apology addressed by the philosopher, Luc Bovens (2008) in his discussion of the apology. His account emphasizes how the apology restores dignity and agency to the one who has been wronged. On Bovens' view, and like Helmreich's, a wrongdoing is a way of disrespecting the victim, specifically by treating her as less than a moral equal, entitled to the same rights as oneself. The failure to regard the victim as a moral equal amounts to the 'offender' placing herself above the victim, looking down on him as inferior. As a result, Bovens argues that there is now a 'respect deficit' between them. The apology restores the equilibrium in respect that ought to obtain between the person who has harmed and the person who has been harmed. This account helpfully shifts the focus of the apology's remedial power from the information conveyed in an apology to the way we relate to the person we have harmed and our intentionality towards them.

No matter how minor or significant the error, apologies have a place in all relationships. Therefore, even a relatively minor 'delinquency' (see Chapter 5) such as being a few minutes late in collecting the patient from the waiting room, for example because we were finishing off a conversation on the phone, requires acknowledgment that we are late, apologizing for this, recognition that we have taken up the time we promised to the patient and the assumption of responsibility for this. Some therapists might understandably be concerned that the apology can inhibit the patient's expression of his anger. Apologies, when they are genuine, tend to de-escalate affect. If this is the case, and we want to argue the merits of not inhibiting the expression of anger, we might ask: how is de-escalation of affect against the patient's best interests? What is the merit in allowing the patient's anger to escalate if the therapist knows that she has provoked it because she was late? Could this be construed as manipulative? There will be different answers to these questions and what matters to ethical practice is that we ask them rather than operate according to established technique. I am of the view that if we have done something wrong, even if it is 'only' being a few minutes late, it is manipulative to not apologize in the service of allowing anger to emerge. If we know that the patient struggles with anger, we can still take this up with him as part of the process, for example acknowledging that an apology does not need to negate the experience and expression of legitimate anger.

Acceptance that harm has been done is integral to a process of reparation. It supports the patient's reality testing and facilitates the process of mourning what was lost or 'stolen'. In his incisive discussion about forgiveness in relation to experiences of trauma, Salman Akhtar discusses how an apology can make a substantive difference through the way that it transposes '. . . the psychic locale of the representations of trauma from the actual to the transitional area of the mind' (2002: 180). Following the apology, Akhtar suggests that . . . 'the trauma begins to get recorded in both the real and the unreal registers of the mind—that is, it acquires a transitional quality. In this realm, it can be more easily played with, looked at from various perspectives, and finally let go' (Akhtar, 2002: 180–181).

The apology thus provides a step in a process of exploration of a range of affects connected with the impact of a trauma or wrongdoing, helping the patient to gradually represent the experience as something that happened in the past and is no longer happening 'now', over and over again. A further benefit of an apology is that it gifts the patient the option of forgiveness (Tylim, 2005). When we forgive another person who has transgressed or harmed us in some minor or more substantive manner, what we are effectively doing, as Akhtar (2002) suggests, is that we act on the past—not by forgetting it but by repeating it in the present and in some way updating it so that it becomes a new past. This process cannot unfold unless the person who has harmed us takes responsibility first, marking that 'it happened'.

Consideration of the function of an apology focuses our attention on the ethical significance of *recognition*, which I touched on in

Chapter 3 when I referred to the harm of misrecognition. An apology is a verbal affirmation that we are seen by the other, that the other recognizes that we have been harmed in a specific way, helping us to understand what happened and why. The therapist who apologizes accepts blame for the injury and in doing so, instead of viewing the patient as an obstacle to her self-interests, he becomes a person with dignity. This validates the patient's beliefs and reality testing, and he can begin or resume a relationship based on these shared values. If the therapist regrets her actions, the patient can take some security in the hope that the therapist will not harm him again. This provides a reason to trust the therapist (Ferenczi, 1933).

Benjamin's (2004) concept of the 'moral third' is central to this discussion and highlights the important function of recognition. The moral third represents

> . . . the principle of interaction . . . that is essential to the recognition process. The moral third may perhaps be best thought of as the principle informing the movement from breakdown to renewal . . . . whereby self and other recreate recognition after breakdown by acknowledging historical responsibility for injury, failure, loss, suffering: the wounds and scars of destructiveness. The process itself, the relational experiences, I think of as thirdness. (2004: 20–21)

The intersubjective focus espoused by clinicians such as Benjamin has a long philosophical tradition dating back to Hegel (1807) who described the unequal power distributions between 'servitude' and 'lordship' culminating in a developmental, historical, and ethical transformation of recognizing the subjectivity of the other. The therapist who can acknowledge her error, who can offer recognition of the consequences of this for the patient, and who can apologize, offers a type of relationship based on mutuality and respect for difference that can advance the analytic process:

> The analyst shoulders responsibility for hurting, even though her action represented an unavoidable piece of enactment. A dyadic system that creates a safe space for such acknowledgment of responsibility provides

the basis for a secure attachment in which understanding is no longer persecutory. . . . If it is no longer a matter of which person is sane, right, healthy, knows best, or the like, and if the analyst is able to acknowledge the patient's suffering without stepping into the position of badness, then the intersubjective space of thirdness is restored. My point is that this step out of helplessness usually involves more than an internal process; it involves direct or transitionally framed communication about one's own reactivity, misattunement, or misunderstanding. (Benjamin, 2004: 32–33)

An apology is thus a fundamentally important process of restitution of the patient's dignity and of his sense of reality and through this it (re)kindles hope in a just and fair world in which he is recognized as having a mind of his own. This becomes possible, as Benjamin suggests '. . . when we are able, as a community, to give up the ideal of being a 'complete container', to surrender to the fact that we survive causing pain' (2009: 442). 'Surviving causing pain' is such a powerful turn of phrase and can be read in two ways. It sensitizes us not only to the inevitability that we will at some stage cause pain to our patients (i.e. a condition of being a therapist is that at some stage we will hurt our patients to ensure our own 'survival',[6] that is, *we* survive *through* causing pain), but it also acts as a reminder that it is possible to recover from the guilt due to the infliction of pain (i.e. we can survive it) as long as we have the humility to see ourselves as flawed and not always acting in the patient's best interests and we have the courage to take responsibility for this.[7,8]

A final consideration concerns *how* we apologize in the context of therapy. An apology, by definition, requires a degree of disclosure. An area of technical divergence amongst the different schools of psychoanalysis is over the function of the therapist's disclosure generally.

---

[6] See also Drozek (2019) on this point.

[7] I do not know what was in Benjamin's mind when she used this turn of phrase. I can only share my reading of it, which may or may not correspond with her explicit intention.

[8] There is some evidence from studies looking at therapist factors associated with better outcomes for patients that effective therapists report making more mistakes than less effective ones and express more 'professional self-doubt' (Heinonen and Nissen-Lie, 2020).

In my view, the vexed technical question about self-disclosure that distinguishes British object-relational schools from intersubjective North American approaches potentially detracts attention away from how we can be present in the analytic relationship and honour the DOC. Whilst I am dubious about the benefits for the patient of therapist self-disclosure as a central therapeutic technique, I am persuaded by the value of moving away from a so-called more 'neutral' style of intervening with the patient that encourages patient and therapist to retreat into their respective solipsistic silos towards a clinical stance that aims to recruit the patient into an explicitly cooperative interaction that cultivates trust, especially when things go wrong. In practice, this means that if I am late for my patient,[9] I do not see any value to the patient of disclosing *why* I was late: it suffices to recognize that I was late, that this is not what I have promised to do, to acknowledge that my lateness has meaning in relation to my breach of the analytic contract and that this breach will hold a very *particular* meaning for each of my patients. I am responsible for acknowledging that 'it happened' and what this means for this patient, which is an acknowledgement in the service of opening exploration, not of shutting it down.

The importance of reparation: The institutional context

Apologies don't exist in a vacuum. Behind every therapist who breaches the ethical code,[10] lies an institution who trained the therapist and who must take a position in relation to one of its members. The analytic culture that supports the development of the *ethical*

---

[9] Of course, being late might occur for reasons that are entirely out of our control (e.g. we are involved in a car accident on the way to work) and as such do not represent an 'error' on our part. In such cases, the apology expresses 'agent regret', that is regret that there has been a breach in the patient's expectation that the session starts on time even though the therapist could not be considered morally responsible for the lateness and the distress this may cause the patient.

[10] Only a minority of these will reach a regulatory threshold that instigates a formal enquiry and I am focusing here on these more substantive breaches.

chóros can only thrive if our training homes practice openness and cooperative interaction that breeds trust, especially when things go wrong.

An apology instigates the process of reparation. Where the breach involves a formal independent investigation, it is important to consider how the institution manages this process both for the patient and for the psychoanalytic community. There are two different kinds of reparation: material as well as symbolic. Much of the difference between traditional court justice, on the one hand, and restorative justice, on the other, derives from the emphasis that the latter places on symbolic reparation. This, it seems, accounts for the greater satisfaction that both victims and offenders feel towards restorative processes as opposed to courtroom trials (Braithwaite, 1999). While material reparation consists almost always in compensation for damage, symbolic reparation is a less visible and more ambiguous process involving social rituals of respect, courtesy, apology, and forgiveness.

The challenge of any professional ethics process is how to constructively take up the position of 'regulator' without this being reduced to the superegoish role of 'the one who sanctions'. As an external observer of professional ethics processes, I have witnessed how this can sometimes mobilize the worst in us: it is all too easy to become the 'moral judge' and to view the colleague who has fallen as very different from us. We feel compelled to clearly demarcate 'us' and 'them' to avert looking at the potential in ourselves for acting in an unethical manner. We may be inclined to banish rather than rehabilitate because what we want to banish is any connection with our own errors or transgressions, however minor, as Glen Gabbard notes:

> What about the time I hugged that patient? Was that sexualized? What about the time I disclosed a highly personal problem to my patient? What about that detailed sexual fantasy I had about my patient? Throwing out the 'rotten apple' is a cleansing process whereby we projectively disavow our own discreditable behavior by depositing it in the transgressing analyst and banishing him or her from the community. (2016: 377)

Drawing on Irvin Goffman's distinction between the 'discredited' and the 'discreditable', Dimen (2021) reminds us that the former carry the stigma of otherness and become convenient repositories for the 'discreditable' parts of ourselves (i.e. the stigma we carry that may not be yet registered as such or perceived by us to be such). For this reason, it behoves us to remain vigilant to the pernicious effects of an overzealous superego. Banishing those who fall foul of the ethical codes may restore a temporary sense of justice or allow us to relegate to the 'them' all that we do not want to countenance or face in ourselves. However, as we know from the rehabilitation of offenders in other fields,[11] the process of rehabilitation is one that can also give the psychoanalytic community the opportunity to learn. This, of course, will not be possible or appropriate in all cases but it needs to be considered as a serious option wherever possible:

> An extreme but not uncommon reaction within a psychoanalytic community is to declare any analyst committing a sexual boundary violation a psychopath. Colleagues on this side of the split may be adamantly opposed to any effort at rehabilitation. Their rage can be so intense that the capacity for objectivity may vanish entirely. Hence the term 'violation' has a double meaning: in addition to violation of the analytic boundary, there has also been a violation of the 'family', the psychoanalytic community. Finally, some colleagues may secretly worry that they were in some way complicit in the transgression because they saw problems but did not speak up. They then take their distance from the offending analyst, making the 'violator' the ultimate 'other'—someone entirely different from the rest of us. (Gabbard, 2016: 375)

At their best, ethics committees and the processes they oversee can restore the 'moral we' (Burka et al., 2019: 262) that is so shattered in the wake of a colleague who commits a boundary violation. The 'moral we', as Burka et al. (2019) suggest, can only be reinvigorated

---

[11] I began my involvement in the helping professions working with criminal offenders and their rehabilitation, so I have to declare that I am especially passionate about rehabilitative processes.

through open dialogue and a willingness to see the colleague who has now become 'other'—no longer part of our moral community—as someone from whom we can also learn through understanding her mistakes.

The challenge is how to create regulatory environments that are rooted in the core values of restorative justice. Restorative justice is concerned with '. . . moral learning, community participation, forgiveness, responsibility, apology, and making amends' (Braithwaite, 1999: 6). Because it underscores the importance of reparation, this kind of justice is thus very aligned with psychoanalytic ideas and values. This invites us to consider the merits of mediated exchanges between a patient and his former therapist where an apology can be safely offered and received, assuming the patient welcomes this opportunity.

Based on his extensive experience of therapists who have been charged with boundary violations, Gabbard (2107) observes that some perpetrators may be incapable of engaging in these forms of reparation, rendering a restorative justice intervention impossible. This we must accept but we can still be open to what may be possible, in some cases at least. Where a criminal offence has taken place, then the law needs to be exercised and no therapist should be treated any differently than any other citizen who commits an offence. If the therapist denies wrongdoing and feels no remorse, it is futile to engage in a reparative process. The therapist's response to an error is key to how an institution proceeds. However, there will be cases where the therapist feels genuine remorse. In such instances we do well to think about how a culture of reparation not only potentially contributes to a process of healing the past but also gives us more hope for the future of our profession.

It is vital to keep in mind that we seem to operate a double standard, as Gentile (2018) aptly observes. We are adept at identifying in our patients the coexistence of areas of high functioning alongside pathology or regressive pulls but we are less receptive to this possibility in ourselves once we become therapists. Therein lie the challenges for us as individual therapists and for our training institutions: how do we straddle contemporaneously being 'behind the couch' and not on it, remain alert to how we can be both helpful and harmful, brilliant in some areas of our analytic selves whilst also capable of making errors and sometimes of minimizing their impact on our patients? We need to work collectively to consolidate organizational cultures that protect patients and support colleagues when things go wrong and the two are, of course, connected. There are two distinguishing features of the organizational culture we should strive to promote in our training homes: it does not idealize psychoanalysis and it is open to scrutiny and dialogue with other disciplines. This is a culture that makes it more possible to come forward and seek help if we are struggling with our work or if we are concerned about a colleague's behaviour. No system is ever perfect but whatever system we have in place for managing the ethics of our discipline, it needs to be transparent, accessible, and fair.

7
Principles in Action

> ... there is an ethical core to psychoanalysis—the psychoanalytic practitioner cannot function adequately without at some point coming to grips with essentially ethical issues, and the psychoanalytic theorist cannot encompass the complexity of the human phenomenon without taking into account the ethical and moral dimensions of man's existence.
> —(Meissner, 1994: 470–471)

Our patients entrust us with their mind, often when they are at their most vulnerable. As therapists we not only have been granted this privileged access to another person's mind, but we also have discretion to make decisions that affect the life and liberty of another person. Ethical dilemmas and risks are inherent to these functions, privileges, and responsibilities. There is a world of difference between armchair ethics and the very real, often urgent pressures that challenge us to make difficult decisions with little time to reflect or debate. Inevitably the examples I share in this chapter are once removed from that real time pressure. However, I hope that they serve as an illustration of how a principled approach, rooted in a widely accepted set of ethical commitments, offers a clearly articulated base from which we can think about our work, even under fire. The five principles I set out in Chapter 3 act as scaffolding for the *ethical chóros* that supports reflection on the factors that we need to take into consideration when we make decisions about how to intervene.

The principled model serves two functions: it helps us to approach broader ethical dilemmas and to monitor individual clinical interventions. In this chapter I will address the former through discussion of the ethical challenges I encountered working with transgender young people and with individuals compelled by the need to change their sexual orientation. I will then illustrate the application of a principled approach to individual interventions, through a commentary on a session transcript. In doing so I hope to further exemplify how ethics, as I use the term in this book, is best conceived of as a process of reflection about how we reach a decision, or of questioning our own clinical practice, that is consistent with the values and purpose of how we understand the nature of psychoanalytic work. This reflective process invites us to move from intuitions to looking at the biases and prejudices that may lie behind our intuitions, looking at the theories we draw on to help us make sense of what we observe, and then move back and forth between these different anchor points. We are striving towards a position of *clinical equipoise*: equally balanced between competing options. This is not as simple as being preference neutral but more a matter of working out whether there are good principled reasons, for instance, to opt for decision/interpretation A or decision/interpretation B.

Using an ethics-based approach to complex clinical dilemmas

Clinical life is not short of examples of ethical dilemmas. A principled approach can help us to tease out the complexity that lies at the core of many ethical debates or struggles and to formulate our unique ethical position in relation to controversial dilemmas. It can assist us in balancing difficult clinical decisions, for example, whether to disclose patient information to a third party, by reminding us to systematically look at the relative costs and benefits of a decision and in relation to the five principles.

As I acknowledged in the Introduction, I am partial to models and frameworks to order my own thinking. In approaching an ethical dilemma in my own mind, I have found it helpful to apply a three-step process: *Specification, Evaluation, and Resolution* (SER). As we engage in this process, which reflects the activation of the *ethical chóros*, we do well to keep in mind that in ethics, there are no right answers.

Different outcomes may be deemed ethical because they are justified by the relative weightings allocated to any of the five principles and given the specifics of each case. The SER model merely reflects a way of systematically working through an ethical dilemma.

Approaching an ethical dilemma always begins with *specification of the ethical problem*, that is what poses the dilemma, what are its specifically ethical challenges, and whom does the problem affect? Understanding the respective interests at play is important. For example, breaching confidentiality to minimize potential harm to the patient or to a third party raises different concerns depending on the 'position' we have in the problem. Is it a question of whether we are ethically justified in intervening and if we don't, are we worried about being liable? Or are we weighing up the options from the patient's perspective (the intrusion of his privacy, the breach of confidentiality, the possible interference with his liberty) and querying what is in his best interests considering the values that we know matter to this patient? The question that taxes us may be something less pressing than whether to breach confidentiality but no less important, for example, whether it is in the patient's best interests to end a therapy that we consider is not supporting psychic change even if the patient is clear that he wishes to continue because it provides support that is of value to him.

Once the problem is identified, we can move to the second step, the *evaluation of the various parameters of the ethical problem*, that is we draw on the five principles and establish which principles are in conflict and subject this to the process of balancing or reflective equilibrium (see Chapters 2 and 3). For example, a therapist may identify that a patient who faces a terminal physical illness is now also depressed and is at risk of suicide. The therapist might instigate an admission to hospital to protect the patient (beneficence) but the patient claims that he has the right to kill himself because he cannot live with the limitations of his physical diagnosis (autonomy). It's clear that in such a scenario one could arrive at quite different positions on what the therapist should do in such a difficult situation depending on our values and commitments to certain ideas about suicide (Cutliffe and Links, 2008). We could question whether depression is a psychiatric illness that undermines autonomy or whether, especially in such a case, one can make a rational decision about dying even if feeling depressed. It may be that the very conceptualization of depression as an illness reflects our commitment to a set of values that are not the only possible values. This is where it is helpful to brainstorm the range of possible arguments for and against the position that comes most naturally to us. We need to be on the alert for the hidden assumption(s) that inform our position and that would benefit from being challenged.

Importantly, part of the process of evaluation involves teasing out fact from value: what are the facts of the case and what are our beliefs and values about these facts? All too often the two become entangled and obscure our capacity to maintain clinical equipoise. Through specifying the problem, we gain some clarity on this but matters of fact and matters of value invariably co-exist in therapy, as they do in life, and our decisions typically comprise both fact and value claims.

Finally, and through the process of reflective equilibrium, we reach the final step, *resolution.* This involves identifying and clarifying the options that flow from the process we have followed through the first two steps of specification and evaluation. In turn, this allows us to spell out a formulation of our ethical response to the identified problem. Now, we can articulate the reasons for why we opted for a particular course of action and how this informs which ethical principle(s) trumps another, thus providing a final layer of review and scrutiny.

I will now focus on two examples of contemporary clinical concern that I have intentionally selected from areas that are controversial and often lead to moral panic, exposing the harms of conservative bias as much as of unthinking political correctness. These examples lend themselves more easily to teasing out the value of a systematic ethical analysis of a clinical dilemma. I have purposefully avoided focusing on more micro dilemmas concerning the therapeutic exchange because these can be found in other textbooks on ethics (e.g. Dewald and Clark, 2007) and because I want to underline the ethical necessity of considering the impact that the therapist's values *inevitably* have on how we think about our patients, their problems, and their aspirations.

Clinical dilemma 1: The ethics of analytic work with under-18-years-old transgender patients

I start with the example of working with young transgender patients because, as I explained in the 'Introduction', it reflects my most recent personal ethical struggle and it illustrates the application of the SER process. I have selected this work because it also reminds us of the interface between the privacy of the analytic relationship and the analytic focus on the patient's internal world and the wider socio-cultural and political realities that inevitably impact on our work, affecting the minds of both patient and therapist alike.

Specification

I started working with individuals who identify as transgender over ten years ago. The ethical dilemma I faced latterly resulted specifically from the rapid increase in referrals of young people who identified as transgender post-puberty with little or no evidence of prior gender dysphoria. My patients (the majority of whom were 12 or over) were all very clear by the time they reached me that they would be happier if they could medically transition. They (mostly) felt that they were seeing me because their parents insisted and not because they perceived themselves to have a problem, besides the distress they experienced associated with the obstacles to transitioning. It was important to specify clearly in my mind that it was this sub-group that raised concerns to avoid the potential risk of generalizing to a heterogeneous category of 'transgender', which is why defining and contextualizing our terms is an essential part of the process of specification. It was clear to me that any conclusions I might draw from my deliberations could only be applicable to this specific group and not to all transgender individuals.

Contemporaneously with the exponential increase in referrals, at a societal level, gender affirmative care was introduced, exposing clinicians to the pressure to 'affirm' the young person's gender of identification without much, if any, exploration. I recognized that I had concerns about how my psychoanalytic focus on exploration of a patient's motives could incur the accusation of being transphobic and of trying to 'convert' my patients to not being transgender.[1] I emphasize this personal concern because in ethical dilemmas there are always different interests at play, and it is helpful to spell these out in one's mind.

Setting aside now the previous considerations, for me the clearest ethical tension arose because of the conflict between the patient's view of what was in their best interests (medical transitioning) and my concern, as I listened to my young patients' experiences and developmental histories, about the possible unconscious drivers that might be exerting an influence on their consciously stated preferences about modifying the body to align it more closely with their gender of identification. I was mindful too that my own understanding of the psychic function of body modification generally (Lemma, 2010, 2022b) made me more likely to question decisions to modify the body and that this might interfere with my capacity to be challenged in my own potentially biased position.

A tension emerged therefore between the importance of supporting the patient's autonomy and the possible entry of psychoanalytic paternalism (i.e. 'I know better than the patient what is best for him'). In this instance, trying to maximize the patient's welfare by helping him to explore his mind and understand if there were unconscious factors driving conscious preference (psychoanalytically informed beneficence) and minimize potential harm (after all, medical

---

[1] The proposed legislation currently debated in the UK in 2022 banning conversion therapy leaves psychoanalytic therapists open to potentially being charged with a new criminal offence of trying to impose 'conversion therapy' if they do not simply affirm the person's self-identification as transgender. At the time of writing this book, this issue remains unresolved.

transitioning carries significant mental and physical health risks) conflicted potentially with patient autonomy. However, it would be more accurate to say that it conflicted with a definition of autonomy denuded of a notion of an unconscious mind, and this needed consideration. Approaching this ethical dilemma psychoanalytically, I was guided by (a) my view that what we want consciously is not necessarily an expression of our autonomy, as we saw in Chapters 2 and 3, and (b) by the age of the patients, which is a relevant consideration with respect to the assessment of autonomy and capacity to consent.

Evaluation

The young people I was working with were typically seeking medical interventions to reduce distress and so, from their perspective, this was about enhancing well-being. As we saw in Chapter 2, well-being has become an important conceptual currency in ethical debates. A fundamental principle of bioethics is that patients should be offered interventions that are in their best interests, which now extends to include interventions that will enhance the psychological and/or social well-being of the person (Savulescu and Kahane, 2011).

The assessment of what constitutes well-being invites us to consider its relationship to a person's values. Values are personal and subjective, sometimes highly idiosyncratic, and subject to change over time, hence decisions about what is best can only be considered on an individual basis. Gender identity is a case in point: how we feel in our body, relative to our individual experience of gender is a subjective state (Wren, 2019), such that it would be very difficult to assign an objective value to it. For some people, the risks associated with medical transitioning, which from my vantage point I identify as 'significant', are nevertheless deemed acceptable to the patient. These considerations helped me to appreciate that from the patient's subjective point of view, I could make a strong case for 'accepting' my young patients' claims about what would make their life go better. This is because a 'good' life, however that is defined (in broad terms and/or in my own personal terms), is not the same as a life that is good *for a particular individual.*

Mindful of the potential interference of my personal and specifically psychoanalytic values, I also had to factor in some 'facts'. Even if we take the patient's privileged access to his mind and his claims about well-being as an essential starting point, we still need to establish that the self-diagnosis is accurate such that the medical interventions are more likely to yield the anticipated benefits. As I reflected on the rise in referrals of under-18-year-olds who present for the first time to services post-puberty identifying as transgender, I was alert to several strands of research and data that invited careful examination of whether the self-certification as transgender might reflect other psychological and/or societal problems (e.g. cross-sex identity in childhood is overwhelmingly predictive of homosexual orientation in adulthood and natal girls are twice as likely to be referred to Gender Identity Development (GID) services, which urges us to investigate the role that social processes may play in the over-representation of girls). It would not be permissible to perform a mastectomy on someone who self-diagnosed as having breast cancer but in fact had bowel cancer. Similarly, performing sex-reassignment surgery on a natal male adolescent who self-identifies as transgender, but may in fact be driven to medically transition due to a conflict about his homosexuality, would not be permissible.

As a psychoanalyst I am of the view that our conscious choices are limited by powerful a priori motivations that can only assist us in decision-making through second-order reflection and evaluation. This process requires time: 'time for self-reflection is not only important psychically, but it is also ethically significant . . . given that the elaboration of unconscious meaning emerges piecemeal over time' (Lemma and Savulescu, 2023: 71). This is one reason why unqualified acceptance of conscious claims can lead to unintended harms. More specifically, affirmation of that which is not in fact the truth is undermining of autonomy and likely to frustrate the patient's interests. If a patient holds a false belief about their condition, his decision about treatment is compromised (Beauchamp and Childress, 2013).

The stage of 'evaluation' thus clarified for me that full autonomy requires not only consideration of medical facts but also the patient must hold deliberated[2] beliefs about his condition, the possible interventions, their risks, and benefits, and importantly about himself and his psychological nature. All these considerations, framed by the tension between competing principles, helped me to focus on the two moral duties I had towards my patients. First, I had to be wary of the moral panic currently surrounding the rise in transgender identification and ensure that this did not undermine my young patients' rights. By 'moral panic' I am referring to the emotional climate framing our reactions to transgender. I have in mind not only the views of those who are gender-critical, but also the views of the transactivists whose concern about injustice and prejudice against transgender people has the potential to quickly escalate into unthinking outrage. Moral panic is inimical to 'thinking well'. Second, I understood that I had a *responsibility* to consider the intrapsychic, social, and/or cultural pressures that might unconsciously influence individual choice about transitioning thereby undermining autonomy and consent.

Let me now illustrate further the clinical and ethical complexity with Sam's case.[3]

Sam, a natal girl, decided to transition from female to male during middle adolescence. Her parents wholeheartedly supported this decision. They said that Sam had always been 'tomboyish'. They were concerned about how depressed he had become, which the parents linked to body dysphoria. Sam scoured the internet for information about his difficulties and found solace in the narratives he read on trans websites. Following three consultations with a specialist gender identity service, Sam was placed on cross-sex hormones and changed his name.

At first Sam's mood improved. He felt very connected to the trans community that he met online, and this eased some of his isolation.

---

[2] I am choosing the term 'deliberated' instead of 'rational', which is more commonly used, because the latter already introduces our values. For example, we may not personally find the belief in God to be rational, but there are people who hold such a belief and who have carefully deliberated on the existence of God.

[3] This fictitious composite case first appeared in Lemma and Savulescu (2021).

However, a year after starting cross-sex hormones, Sam took a serious overdose and was admitted to an in-patient facility. It was only at this point that he was referred for psychological help.

During the process of psychotherapy that ensued, it quickly emerged that Sam's much older brother had died unexpectedly when Sam was still a very young child. The brother had been a strong presence in the family and Sam thought that his mother preferred him. He felt that his mother had never really recovered from this tragic loss. He conveyed how he had tried hard to please her as best he could and how upset he was when he felt unable to assuage her loss.

As a younger child, Sam did not recall wanting to be a boy, but he was clear that he had taken a strong interest in more typically 'male' sports (like Sam knew that the brother had done) and preferred playing with boys, which had alienated him from the girls at school. The parents had told Sam that he had expressed a strong wish to have been born a boy when he was at primary school. Sam had no recollection of saying this to them but at the start of therapy he was nevertheless adamant that this was how he had always felt.

When Sam eventually decided that he wanted to transition, the parents were very supportive. Sam recalled feeling closer to them than ever before. He had the impression that they were happier overall, especially his mother. Over time in the therapy, it became clear that, as far as Sam was concerned, the decision to transition had facilitated a closeness between him and his mother that he had always longed for.

The parents appeared to have been very invested in Sam's decision, even hurrying the process of starting hormones and attributed the suicide attempt exclusively to Sam's gender dysphoria. The suicide attempt accelerated their belief that Sam should undergo sex reassignment surgery at the earliest opportunity. Yet Sam's own account of the events leading to the suicide attempt did not appear to be evidently connected to gender dysphoria. Rather, the suicide attempt seemed to have been triggered by Sam's feelings of distress and anger after the parents missed an important celebratory event in Sam's life because it coincided with the anniversary of his brother's death, which they always marked, and around which Sam often felt very uncomfortable.

The brother's 'ghost' dominated the family's collective psyche; for example, the brother's bedroom had been preserved and Sam was often compared to the brother. Sam had very little memory of his brother and at times he resented the brother's ongoing presence and preference in the mother's mind. Sam was tortured by guilt that he had survived his brother as well as guilt about his resentment towards him for taking up the parents' mental space which Sam wanted to claim for himself.

Sam had grown up in his brother's shadow engulfed by the parents' unresolved grief. In the context of therapy, Sam came to understand that the only way that he had felt he could be 'seen' by his parents was to effectively become their 'son' through transitioning. Yet, despite starting medical transitioning, Sam was soon confronted with the actual impossibility of replacing his brother. This became painfully clear to him when his parents cancelled their attendance at a celebratory event for Sam because it coincided with the anniversary of the brother's death. Sam's suicide attempt was another way in which he used his body to recall his parents' attention to his existence and needs. But their misreading, as it were, of why he had tried to kill himself, left Sam feeling alienated from them and confused about whether he should seek sex reassignment surgery.

As the family dynamics were consciously articulated, gender identity receded in Sam's mind as either the problem or the solution and the focus turned instead to Sam's distress and grievance towards his parents for what he had experienced as their neglect of his needs. Awareness of how the unresolved family grief and his own longing to be the replacement son had informed his transgender identification enabled him to make informed choices about the best next steps for him.

Clearly not all individuals who express the wish to transition are motivated by underlying psychological problems, as was the case for Sam. Yet Sam's case underscores the complexity of assessing autonomy when we factor in systemic and intrapsychic unconscious pressures on self-perception and identity development. Sam appeared to have been driven primarily by a wish to claim a space in his parents' minds (especially his mother's) that he felt was occupied by his deceased brother. He unconsciously resolved to do this by identifying as a boy and then asking to transition so that he could replace his brother. Even though the family was not consciously co-ercing Sam to change gender, it could be argued that there was an un-conscious investment in supporting the gender transition to reclaim their lost son. Systemic pressures can thus potentially function to en-force conformity to unconscious needs that act against the person's best interests. Sam's case illustrates the operation of the complex relationship between external and internal pressures on decision making. The external pressure, however, is not recognized as such consciously by Sam. It is unreflectively internalized and takes on a life of its own in the idiosyncratic prerogatives of his internal world, not least his own unconscious longing to be loved by his parents and to replace his brother and the guilt this provokes.

Sam's case can, and indeed should be, countered by cases that re-veal that transitioning is, all things considered, better for the person. As we go through the stage of 'evaluation', it is essential to consider cases that provide a counterargument. In my own practice I could draw on such examples (see Section 3). These provided important reminders that medical transitioning can enhance well-being and be an expression of autonomy. However, the fact that transitioning can be a positive outcome for some, is not an argument against a thor-ough exploration of the motivations for wanting to transition so as to ensure that the decisions taken can be said to be substantially auton-omous and substantially independent from controlling forces.

Resolution

The process of evaluation of the ethical dilemma enabled me to artic-ulate my overall ethical position with respect to my young patients. This provided an important anchor as I approached my work in what has, unfortunately, become a contested area of clinical practice. My deliberations led me to the following internal position: a decision to transition cannot be an instantiation of autonomy if it is based on a false or partial narrative that prevents the person from accessing the help and resources appropriate to the state that undermines their well-being. The individual's *current* wishes, no matter how strongly felt, are not always a reliable indicator of what will enhance well-being. My ethical deliberations with cases like Sam's thus led me to specify an analytic position that supports the ethical necessity of exploration to protect the young people I was seeing from exercising 'autonomy' that I understood to be only surface deep. In other words, the problem is not transitioning per se, but the psychic position from which we arrive at that decision. Unqualified acceptance of conscious claims can reduce the individual's options and autonomy if it deprives them of an opportunity to explore the possible unconscious meaning of their transgender identification which, in turn, might lead them to consider options other than medical transitioning.

Resolving an ethical dilemma and finding a position that feels coherent brings some relief, but the essence of ethics is remembering that no two cases are alike. The ethical position that was appropriate in Sam's case was specific to him. The general principles that I articulated in response to this work have potential validity as an overall framework but they require testing out against other cases that might yet have a different outcome. I will now illustrate this point through Kay's case.[4]

In my work with some patients who are intent on modifying the body, this decision appears to be very clearly connected to traumatic events in childhood. The psychoanalytic inclination is to address the trauma in the hope that this will relieve the pressure to act on the body. Addressing the trauma is essential. However, in some cases, I have been challenged to consider that insight may not be sufficient to render obsolete the need to modify the body. Or, to frame this differently thus exposing and then shedding my own psychoanalytic prejudices, we might say that insight provides the patient with a foundation for determining whether the modification of the body still offers something of value to them—a value that can only be assessed relative to the individual's value system and current psychological needs.

---

[4] This section is adapted from Lemma (2022a). Kay's case is a fictitious composite case drawing on recurring dynamics observed across several patients with whom I have worked and reflects how I have understood these patients' presentation.

Kay first came to see me in her mid-twenties because she wanted to undergo a double mastectomy to align her natal female body with her subjective sense of transgender identity. Kay was depressed and struggling in many aspects of her life. She detailed a long history of significant discomfort in her body, feeling that since she was a child, she had disliked her 'feminine form'. She identified as gender fluid, was comfortable with the feminine pronoun, but said that she had always wished that she had been born a boy. Over time Kay became insightful about the origins of her bodily discomfort and was able to connect it to traumatic events in her childhood. In therapy she explored the motivations for her wish for surgery, recognizing that some people might view it as an extreme measure but for her it felt 'right'.

For Kay, the image of herself with a flat chest made her feel better— she felt more confident and truer to who she felt herself to be. She could see that if she had not had the childhood she had, she might have felt differently, but she thought this was beside the point: her past had shaped not only what she did not like (her breasts) but also what she preferred (to be flat chested and to look androgynous). She was clear about the risks of surgery and that she could potentially regret this, but for her these were risks worth taking.

After over two years of twice weekly psychotherapy, Kay resolved to pursue a double mastectomy. Kay said that she had no doubts that pursuing surgery was the right decision for her. She was aware, she said, that I seemed committed to helping her to go on exploring this decision but as far as she was concerned, she had spent two years doing this and her decision remained the same. She said that she now felt better overall. She was satisfied that we had addressed her motivations from every possible angle. I detected some exasperation on her part with what she (accurately) perceived to be my bias towards more exploration.

As I reflected on my work with Kay, I was starkly confronted with how I had been in the sway of my need to rescue her from a decision that I evidently struggled with. Kay challenged me to view her decision to purse surgery as denoting what I can best describe as a *cognisant adaptation* to who she felt herself to be and aspired to be given her history. Kay was meaningfully connected to her history of trauma and how this shaped her relationship to her body. Even so, in her mind the representation of her flat-chested body was one that made her feel safe and confident and it was therefore aspired to. The projected bodily representation of the body-to-be (a flat-chested body that she felt would not signal 'sexy woman', but 'strong') rather than the 'body that holds the memory' (a visibly female body, for Kay) had been an essential and adaptive defence to the traumatic circumstances in early childhood.

This type of clinical presentation distinguishes itself from a traumatic adaptation where the patient is unaware of the ongoing impact of the trauma on his decisions. By contrast, Kay illustrates how a patient can have insight into the links between the trauma and the desire to modify the body (i.e. is not in denial) and yet resolves to pursue the modification of the body. Another patient might well have chosen to persevere with more exploration, but the fact that Kay chose surgery, cognisant of her own history and of the risks associated with her choice, challenges us to recognize that an individual can make an informed choice about an imagined bodily form that bolsters feelings of safety and preserves adaptation in the outside world such that surgery is, for them, a price worth paying. Despite the reduction of the original conflict that brought the traumatic adaptation into being, patients such as Kay remind us that defences that were once essential to psychic survival may persist and support a good-enough adaptation in external reality, all things considered (Joffe and Sandler, 1968).

If my work with Kay had stopped at the time that she resolved to pursue surgery, I suspect that I would still be wondering if Kay had made the best possible decision for her or whether I had simply not been able to help her enough. However, Kay stayed in therapy for several years post-surgery. I could observe that the surgery did help her to feel at home in her body and accommodate its history. She was able to finally enjoy a close sexual relationship, be more comfortable in group situations, and she developed a fulfilling professional career. Within bioethics, autonomy is often equated with informed consent about one's medical care, principally the right to refuse treatment (which was historically necessary, given the strong paternalism that

pervaded health care). However, as we saw in Chapter 2, we understand autonomy nowadays in a deeper sense: to respect someone's
autonomy is to recognize the person as capable of shaping his life
and the kind of person he wants to be. On this richer account, respect for patient autonomy includes a presumption that we should
always consider a patient's desires, values, feelings, and plans when
considering what he wants from a therapeutic process.

My encounter with Kay was a sobering reminder that what we
privilege in our view of what makes a life go well may be at odds with
the patient's view. Notwithstanding important nuances across theorists, the analytic notion of health is rooted in the importance of
bearing frustration, of accepting our ultimate helplessness, and the
reality of loss. This orients the therapist in a very particular way, for
example, to requests for modifying the body. From this psychoanalytic vantage point, enhancement, and modification of the healthy
natal body, in whatever form, can only be viewed suspiciously at first.
Whilst a patient may well be deluded or in the grip of an omnipotent
organization when they seek to modify the body, this is not invariably so. We live in a pluralistic society in which the idea of the good
life cannot be assumed to be identical for everyone, and recognition
of this fact is ethically significant. Changing the body does not necessarily entail denial or omnipotent triumph over the internal object
relationships. On the contrary, some people may avail themselves of
the greater and more accessible opportunities nowadays to modify
the body, altering sex characteristics for purposes of identity exploration or 'creative transfiguration' (Ashley and Ells, 2018).[5] In other
words, they may seek to enhance the form of their embodiment in a
way that better suits their sense of who they are and of their values
(Zohny, Earp, and Savulescu, 2022). For patients like Kay, changing
the body is a way of adapting to one's history, not denying it, and
therapy helps the patient to reach a stage when meaningful consent
to the medical intervention is possible.

---

[5] The age of the person electing to undergo such bodily transfigurations is nevertheless a significant ethical consideration.

Autonomous functioning, as we have seen, requires that we have access to a realistic appraisal of the internal and external influences that bear on what we think we want for ourselves (Lemma and Savulescu, 2023). This evaluation requires access to both conscious and unconscious 'facts' (i.e. possible *unconscious* drivers). Once these unconscious influences become objects of conscious reflection, we can take steps to reduce or accommodate their effect on our behaviour and decisions. If medical transitioning is a reasonable option for the patient, the patient may in the end opt for it, even if it is less than the best course of action. In this sense, autonomy may trump best interests (Lemma and Savulescu, 2023). Each patient deserves and has a right to a journey to identify what is most likely to promote their well-being. This way of situating ourselves as we listen requires that we are less interested in identifying whether the patient has a disorder (as though the question could be objectively decided, that is, without appeal to potentially disputable value judgments) or whether what he seeks conforms with our psychoanalytically expected view of 'normal' functioning.[6] It is essential to engage with each patient singularly and without a pre-ordained outcome at the back of our minds. At its best that is how psychoanalysis is oriented. But I have observed in myself and in colleagues that decisions by the patient to change the so-called given body can be provocative, confronting the therapist with a tension between her values and definition of psychic health and the patient's desires and values. The risk is then that the words, values, and intentions of the patient in the service of articulating a viable identity are not given the same weight as those of the therapist. This potentially exposes the patient to epistemic injustice (see Chapter 3).

An ethical struggle creates opportunities for clarification and impacts future work. My experience with transgender patients, and the ethical tension it created within me, prompted me to reflect more broadly about what position may be most helpful when working in

---

[6] See Roache and Savulescu (2018) for a clear and challenging discussion of the welfarist view of psychiatric diagnosis.

this highly complex and emotional area for both patient and therapist. I have emphasized the importance of treating each case individually but this does not preclude an attempt to find an overarching internal ethical position. No doubt, other colleagues would reach different conclusions or positions. For me, the analytic journey with patients who feel the need to modify their bodies through surgery, whether they see themselves as transgender or not, has focalized that the primary aim of analytic work lies not in any predetermined outcome congruent with the therapist's definition of psychic health, but in the protection of the analytic space so that the patient can discover the unconscious determinants of his choice(s). This provides the foundations for a more realistic assessment of whether his decision to modify the body and the risks/costs associated with it is one worth taking. In turn, this enhances the patient's autonomy in relation to the choice (or not) to modify the body.

So where does this leave us in terms of our responsibility to our patients? Our ethical responsibility, I suggest, is limited to the following. First, we must protect the integrity of the process that facilitates psychoanalytic exploration, with due attention to the operation of unconscious factors in both parties. As we saw in Chapter 3, this requires us to be committed to an ongoing process of self-questioning. Second, and related to the first point, we must try to be clear about the ethical position with which we side with respect to any number of issues so that we can bracket this and protect the analytic space for the patient to elaborate his own mind/position, which may well be at odds with ours. Patient preference and his own conception of the good life should be central to the analytic process or else we veer in the direction of a version of paternalism that I personally struggle to defend. This does not mean that we must agree with the patient or withhold our understanding because it differs. It primarily means that we share our thoughts mindful that our perspective is not the final arbiter of what the patient should do. It is an offering that the patient may or may not find helpful. However, we need to recognize that our words carry a particular transferential weight and have greater impact by virtue of our professional role such that what we say is never neutral.

Clinical dilemma 2: The ethics of conversion therapy

In this second example, I want to illustrate the importance of taking a step back from the immediacy of the affective heat that some clinical dilemmas evoke—which is, in my view, a primary function of the *ethical chóros* (i.e. we step back into this self-reflective space)—and look at the problem more dispassionately. This can allow us to discern important nuances that, in turn, generate further questions. I have opted to address another controversial topic because such topics tend to provide the most fertile ground for examining the relative benefits of applied ethical analysis.

At the time of writing this book in early 2022, the UK government is seeking to introduce very important and much overdue legislation banning conversion therapy. Conversion therapy refers to any psychological or medical intervention offered with the intention of changing a person's sexual orientation or their gender identity. Although these practices vary in the methods they use, they are united by their belief that being gay, lesbian, bisexual, or transgender are 'conditions' that should be cured. Legislation to ban this practice can only be seen to be a very positive step. I have been personally unambiguously supportive of these changes in the public domain. It is essential that society regulates the practice of conversion therapy to protect vulnerable individuals and the right to express one's sexual preferences and gender identity without fear of intimidation or discrimination. However, in the service of illustrating the ethical complexity that may lie beneath what seems like a self-evidently good change of practice, let's consider the following hypothetical example of Mr A.[7] Through this I hope to (a) illustrate how considerations about the principle of autonomy might make us pause before

---

[7] This is a fictitious case informed by my clinical experiences with people who were referred to me because they were specifically troubled by sexual conflicts especially around the requirement to be celibate due to being Catholic priests, for example, and/or they reported feeling conflicted about their sexual orientation, and a very small minority contemplated conversion therapy. For the absence of doubt, my work *never* involved offering conversion therapy or recommending it, but I draw on the experience to illustrate the internal steps of thinking through an ethical dilemma.

agreeing unreservedly with an argument in favour of an *unqualified* ban on the practice of conversion therapy and (b) highlight the importance of 'balancing' that I described in Chapter 2.

Mr A was a priest. He was adamant that he wanted to undertake conversion therapy to change his sexual orientation. He viewed this as in his best interests. This was very challenging for me because of own my personal views on conversion therapy (i.e. a practice that should be stopped) and his request stymied me: what was an ethical response to such a request? Psychoanalytically speaking the answer may seem simple and obvious: we are not here to direct the patient; rather our task is to enable self-reflection that might help the patient with his decision and to examine the unconscious drivers that support the patient's experience of his sexuality as ego-dystonic. But I imagine that, like me, some therapists would approach listening to this man's request with some prejudgement about conversion therapy and through which their listening would be filtered.

My starting presumption is that conversion therapy is an unethical practice and that it would never be permissible for a therapist to support such a request. Even if the request originates from the patient, our responsibility is to invite the patient to examine his reasons for wanting to undergo such an intervention, just as I argued earlier in relation to requests for medical transitioning. In other words, our role is to create the conditions for examining the meaning of such a request and not reinforcing any homophobic views that the patient may potentially harbour towards himself.

A merit of applied ethics is that it pushes us to think about the counterarguments to any position we subscribe to. For example, does my presumption that conversion therapy is unethical imply that it could *never* be morally permissible? This is an interesting and important conundrum to explore because it is only when we can be receptive to a range of positions that we can minimize the intrusion of our own values. In order to flesh out ethical dilemmas, ethicists turn to hypothetical scenarios or what are referred to as 'thought experiments'. The idea is to look at scenarios that need not reflect what actually *is*. By looking at '. . . *but what if ...*' hypothetical scenarios it becomes possible to tease out the basic principles that drive our ethical position on any manner of issues. So, in this spirit, let's imagine that conversion therapy is *both safe and effective* (which we know *not* to be the case in reality). However, *if* this were the case, how might we think about how to help Mr A, the priest, who approaches us about seeking conversion therapy to change his sexual orientation? Do we think that it could ever be morally permissible to offer this type of intervention, if it were safe and effective? I am not inviting you to consider whether you would ever provide it, but simply to reflect on how you might think about whether it could *ever* be in Mr A's best interests. I will address this through looking at how the ethical question raised by Mr A's case compares with that raised by the specifics of another patient, Mr B, who was forced to undergo conversion therapy.

Let's start with Mr A who urgently wanted to 'convert' so that he could pursue his vocation without struggling with his homosexual orientation, which he found debilitating. For him, the idea of being homosexual and a priest created intense conflict. However, if he imagined leaving the clergy, Mr A's life lost meaning and purpose: he could not imagine a life in which he was not a priest but neither could he tolerate a life as a priest with homosexual longings. He was clear that his position in the church did not depend on undergoing conversion therapy. Nevertheless, Mr A felt that being homosexual was to be 'disordered', he knew that this view was prevalent in his religious community, and this view of himself was ego-dystonic. His enlightened bishop had tried to dissuade Mr A from conversion therapy and encouraged instead the route of living with his conflict. Moreover, Mr A had not been forced to become a priest and he was not being forced to convert his sexual orientation either. But to do this job, Mr A had to manage the knowledge that within his own faith system homosexuality was understood by many to be 'sinful' or a 'disorder' and he needed to address his own internal conflicts around his sexuality.

Let us now turn to the case of Mr B, a young Asian man, who had hidden his homosexuality from his family. When his parents found him a potential wife, he refused to marry her, finally admitting to them that he was gay. His parents reacted angrily, shamed him, and asked him to move out of the family home where he had been residing. They refused to see him unless he had regular meetings with a 'community healer' to 'cure' him of his homosexual longings. Mr B eventually agreed to this because he did not want to be alienated from his family and community. Mr B was under enormous external pressure to 'give up' his homosexual identity, which was ego-syntonic, in order to be accepted by his family. After several sessions with the healer, Mr B took an overdose, which he survived, and was only then referred to therapy.

Compared to Mr A, Mr B was more evidently under *external* pressure to conform to the norms espoused by his family and cultural community. We might say that he was coerced by his family to see the healer. If he did not agree to see the healer (option A), then he was exposed to option B (you cannot live here with us and be loved by us); and A and B were the only options open to him. This is the essence of coercion (Nozick, 1969). By contrast, Mr A was not being pressured by an external force to choose between being a priest or not being a priest. He had taken up a 'job' as a priest fully aware of the conditions and his bishop was advising him to find a way of reconciling himself with his sexuality. Yet Mr A still wanted to undergo conversion therapy.

As we have seen, an important ethical consideration when working with a patient who has to make significant decisions about his life, is to assess whether he is functioning autonomously. Mr B's agreement to convert does not meet the requirement of an autonomous choice: Mr B is coerced by clear family and community pressures. The situation is more complex in Mr A's case. He was clear that he prioritized being a priest over other values, such as the importance of being true to his sexual orientation, and he viewed his sexuality as a liability but there was no evidence of coercion from external sources. Psychoanalytically speaking, we might wonder whether Mr A is under the sway of *unconscious coercion* perpetrated by his own (unconscious) internal homophobe against his homosexual self and that it is this that drives him to want to subject himself to conversion therapy. If this was the case, his decision to undergo conversion therapy could not be said to be autonomous.

For the sake of argument, let's imagine that this possibility is explored in the therapy and Mr A can acknowledge his own internal conflicts around being homosexual. However, this continues to trouble him, it is a source of pain, and he feels that, on balance, given that there is an effective way of stopping the pain by undergoing conversion therapy, then this is his best option.

In this case, and always assuming that conversion therapy was safe and effective, we could argue that if Mr A did find a conversion therapist, it would be morally permissible to offer him this option because (a) his sexual orientation is experienced as significantly incongruent with other important values that promote his well-being, (b) this causes suffering (maleficence), (c) Mr A has the chance to explore this in therapy and remains of the view that, on balance, conversion therapy is better for him, and (d) he is competent to make a rational autonomous choice (autonomy). Even if we were to now step back into reality where we know that it is *not* a safe and effective intervention, we could still argue that if Mr A was not being coerced, and he understood that there was no evidence that conversion therapy was either safe or effective, Mr A nevertheless has the right to still pursue it.

Even so, this is not an open and shut case. Ethics urges us to think further. It could be argued that Mr A cannot be considered free to choose to have conversion therapy because this 'choice' is made in the context of, and partly in response to, a religious system that perpetuates a view of homosexuality that is wrong and that itself creates harms. Supporting conversion therapy, even if at Mr A's insistent request, and even if it were a safe and effective intervention, would reinforce prejudice rather than challenge it.

The principle of beneficence urges us to promote individual patient welfare without becoming complicit in the perpetuation of unjust social norms (Earp, 2014). When we are faced with harms caused by discrimination of any kind, we have two potentially competing moral obligations: one is to prioritize social change, the other is to minimize the harm to those affected whilst awaiting the broader scale of social change to be implemented. Moreover, the hypothetical availability of an effective and safe conversion therapy does not protect against its use to coerce people into it. Any intervention that could influence a person's identity, and that could be abused, requires tight regulation and protocols to ensure that if it is used, diversity is protected.

To return to Mr A. Even if we might eventually get to a stage in society in which belonging to his religious group would not involve exposing himself to a prejudiced view of homosexuality, given the time it takes to eradicate societal prejudices, this might be unlikely to happen in the short or medium term of Mr A's life. So, whilst supporting social change is praiseworthy, it might be supererogatory to expect people in Mr A's situation to continue to struggle with such conflicts whilst social changes are embedded. How could we justify asking Mr A to wait for society to change and deprive him of an intervention that would relieve him of his distress given that in our hypothetical example, conversion therapy is effective? This could be, all things considered, beneficial for him, even if only as a way of avoiding an experience of alienation or conflict in a prejudiced enclave of society. We could continue to argue for and against, but I will not dwell further on the specifics of this hypothetical example. Suffice to say that I hope both this example and the dilemmas raised by work with young transgender patients illustrate three key ethical points that bear on our everyday work as therapists.

First, I dwelt on the hypothetical example of Mr A to illustrate how there is no 'right' position: it is possible to convincingly argue the case for and against the decision to pursue conversion therapy for someone like Mr A, assuming it was a safe and effective intervention. Even when we know that it is not safe and effective, if this is the path that Mr A wants to pursue in the fullness of the knowledge of the risks and its function in his psychic economy, then we could argue that he has a right to do so. The ethical position we assume in relation to any dilemma thus always benefits from consideration of the other side of the argument. Ethical enquiry should make us feel uncomfortable so as to ensure that we robustly challenge the first line of response that seems morally correct. The five principles frame these deliberations. Some of the principles will be more salient than others depending on the case, but the framework acts as a reminder of all the dimensions that we should consider before coming to any conclusions.

Second, working ethically requires us to remain alert to how our analytic focus on the patient's internal world always unfolds in an external social context, which is one of several relevant considerations in our understanding of what may be in the patient's best interests. Ignoring such external factors, I suggest, is not just clinically but also ethically dubious. The internal world of the patient does not exist in a vacuum: it is in a constant dynamic interplay with external forces. Ethical debate pushes us to stay engaged with the social world and its exigencies, limitations, and opportunities, which as we know are not evenly distributed. Ethics, in my view, keep psychoanalysis on its toes, so that its traditional emphasis on the internal world is not diminished but enhanced through the tension created by the necessary dialogue with ethical principles that bring into focus the complex, intersected realities of the external world.

Third, and related to the second point, it is essential that we are willing to consider *whose* values are operative in steering the work in an analytic dyad. If as a therapist, I find the notion of conversion therapy abhorrent—even if it were safe and effective—because I believe that we should live in a world where sexual orientation should not make anyone feel inferior or different in a negative sense, how do we steer this value around the patient's value system or the pain he is experiencing and which frames his decisions, if it differs markedly from our own priorities or values? Over the course of therapy, and sometimes prompting the search for therapy, is the patient's preoccupation with some crucial decisions he needs to make. As I have suggested before, our commitment to neutrality cannot make us immune to the implicit influence that our values have on the questions we ask or don't ask or on the interpretations we consider to be important, all of which steer the patient towards exploring some possibilities and foreclosing others.

Monitoring the ethics of everyday practice

Fortunately, ethical dilemmas do not occur every day. However, the interventions that we make with our patients are an everyday occurrence. The outcome of psychotherapy is now the subject of much research and is measured against outcomes that are (more or less) quantifiable. I am interested here not in how we evaluate our practice in terms of overall outcomes, but in terms of the ethics embedded in the interventions we make with our patients or that we omit to make. I suggest that the five principles can also be applied systematically to support our ongoing monitoring of our interventions.

By way of an example, let's look at the clinical decision to 'remain silent' as we listen to a patient who becomes visibly distressed near the end of a session. Using the model that I have been advocating, any decision about how to intervene, in this instance 'to remain silent', can be evaluated against the following five questions. As I am not discussing a specific patient, I am only illustrating for now the range of the questions that keep us focused on the ethics of our work. It is important to keep in mind that we can never be absolute in the rightness or wrongness of our answer, but we can have stronger or weaker reasons for supporting our decision(s) on how we intervene at any given moment.

1. *Non-maleficence—Does it harm the patient?* Will the silence result in the patient feeling abandoned at a time of acute distress and amplify the subjective experience of distress? If this is a recurrent dynamic and there is a concern about colluding and being drawn into rescuing the patient, is the patient's state of arousal such that silence can be of benefit or might it instead escalate arousal and leave the patient too raw just before the session end and hence be potentially harmful?

2. *Beneficence—Does it benefit the patient?* Will the silence be difficult to bear, and might cause temporary amplification of distress (i.e. a short-term harm), but might this be balanced out if it also contributes to a helpful elaboration of the experience

of abandonment that benefits the patient longer term and thus furthers his best interests? Will the silence be experienced as implicit confirmation from the therapist that she thinks the patient can manage his pain and does not need her intervention, thus strengthening the patient's experience of more autonomous functioning? The question about beneficence therefore needs to be considered alongside the earlier question about maleficence. It requires balancing risks and potential benefits.

3. *Autonomy—Does it show respect for the patient and his right to make decisions for himself?* Will silence support the patient's autonomy through the experience that the therapist does not rush in with verbal reassurance or an interpretation, say about dependency, but instead implicitly trusts in the patient's capacity to elaborate the experience of abandonment and contains it through the silence? Or does the silence undermine autonomy because if the patient becomes affectively disorganized by the therapist's silence, he will be less able to mentalize, and this impacts adversely on autonomous functioning.

4. *Veracity—Am I being truthful?* This question concerns our intentionality. Why am I being silent? Is it because I believe that it is in the patient's best interests, or am I simply not sure what I think? Or am I too tired and that is why I say nothing, hiding behind the accepted norm that silence is helpful to encourage free association, even though in this instance it is simply not helpful? Or am I following what I think my supervisor would say I should do, and hence I want to ensure I am approved of, rather than focusing on what this patient needs right now?

5. *Justice—Are there consequences in the wider community or with respect to fairness?* Consideration of fairness, which rests on the ability to appreciate differences between people, is relevant to whether silence may be contraindicated with a patient whose cognitive difficulties or neurodiversity, for example, mean that the impact of a silent response disadvantages him in a very specific way. This may be because he may not understand why the

therapist is silent and may need more active input from the therapist to process a difficult affect.

We could apply this five questions template to any intervention. Its merit is that it encourages us to consider different angles on why we make an intervention and whether it is in the service of helping the patient rather than driven by another agenda. This is an especially important consideration during training when our relationships to supervisors and our wish to please them may lead us to intervene in particular ways because that is what is expected by them rather than what is needed by the patient. To this end, I now turn to the interpretation of transference—a mainstay of analytic technique— which provides a good example of an intervention that we may make at times because that is what we are taught is the essence of a psycho-analytic approach rather than because it is necessarily most helpful to the patient (Lemma, 2013).

The earlier trend in psychoanalysis towards caricatured, excessive interpretation of the 'you mean me' variety of transference interpretation[8] has given way to an increasingly sophisticated and differenti-ated approach. Nowadays careful attention is paid to the importance of the timing and frequency of interpretations, of the moment-by-moment assessment of the patient's tolerance for a transference focus, and of the way transference dynamics may be most helpfully approached in an interpretation (e.g. the use of therapist-centred or analyst-centred interpretations (Steiner, 1993). Notwithstanding this more considered approach to working in the transference, we nevertheless accord it a privileged position in our conceptualizations of what promotes change, and hence what we think we should be doing with a patient, with the attendant risk that when we are *not* taking up the transference, we may feel that we are not working psy-choanalytically. In turn, this can make it harder to examine the value

---

[8] When I refer to working in the transference, I am using the term in a Kleinian sense: the transference is more than just a repetition of the patient's patterns of relating to significant fig-ures in the past; rather, it is primarily about the patient's internal world—his world of uncon-scious phantasy—as it becomes manifest in his total attitude to the therapist and to the analytic setting.

of other interventions in an unprejudiced way and may interfere with our capacity to prioritize the intervention that most benefits the patient in a given moment.[9]

In my experience, interpreting the transference is the most mutative intervention with some patients much of the time, with many patients *some* of the time, and with a minority it needs to be used very sparingly, if at all. In other words, it is a fundamentally important technique, but it is not the *only* effective route to psychic change for all patients. In putting the interpretation of the here-and-now transference 'on the ethical couch', as it were, I am extending an invitation to critically examine our belief that working in the transference is the holy analytic grail. Any type of 'belief-led' way of working can have an insidious effect on our work, which at its best should operate in the spirit of unprejudiced enquiry rather than make us pursue 'overvalued ideas' (Britton and Steiner, 1994), which is an ethical tipping point.

I would now like to share some brief clinical material of my own to provide a snapshot of the kind of internal and inherently ethical work we strive to engage in when considering whether and how to intervene.[10]

> Mr C—a successful businessman in his late thirties—cancelled his Monday and Tuesday sessions due to being ill. Such cancellations were a common part of his relational repertoire: he inched closer to his objects only to then withdraw. With a string of carefully choreographed long-distance relationships to his name, Mr C found himself seeking analysis because he was preoccupied with death and suffered terrible nightmares, which led to a fear of going to sleep.
>
> The most immediate trigger for seeking help had been the death of his mother, who had raised him alone after the father's death when he

---

[9] Indeed, the range of what we actually do in our consulting rooms is much broader than 'official' clinical theory (Tuckett, 2008; Jimenez, 2009). I am sure we will recognize that we all say and do a range of helpful things that would not be defined as 'interpreting the transference', such as making an observation about patterns apparent in the patient's external relationships, asking questions to clarify meaning or to encourage further elaboration of associations, staying silent, laughing with the patient, interpreting his dreams.

[10] This detailed clinical material was first published in Lemma (2013).

was seven. Theirs had been a close relationship, and he had relied on his mother extensively, but he also experienced her as intrusive, demanding, and suffocating. The death of his mother destabilized him—he felt suddenly alone and lost, revisiting the early loss of his father too.

Mr C had always struggled to form intimate relationships, fearing a repeat of the seductive yet claustrophobic experience with his mother. Despite these profound anxieties Mr C nevertheless also longed to have a relationship—a longing that was coloured by his memory of a father who had been quietly present and whose loss had been devastating for him, exposing Mr C to a mother who needed him at all costs to assuage her own pervasive anxiety. Eighteen months into our work he had nevertheless managed to settle into a more stable relationship with a woman he was now contemplating living with, though this prospect had thrown him, once again, into crisis.

In the session in question, the third of the week, Mr C began by saying he was feeling overwhelmed by the 'long list' of decisions he had to make. He was considering buying a bigger property to move in with his partner, but this raised the question of starting a family, which he simply did not want to think about. He accused his partner of putting pressure on him to face his procrastination. All he wanted, he said emphatically and irritably, was some 'peace of mind'. He said that his partner reminded him on these occasions of his mother and how she had 'kept him on a leash'—an expression that he had used before to describe how he felt his mother had always kept him in line, telling him what to do, interfering in his personal affairs.

As I listened, I sensed that he was warning me I should not get him to think about this external situation or his missed sessions, that I should instead simply listen and not add to his already 'long list'. This was a not unfamiliar instruction: Mr C was very controlling of his objects, and this was a prominent experience in the transference.

Mr C went on to say that he felt there was no space for him in his life and then he mentioned that the one thing he had enjoyed doing—in fact the only thing that had made him feel better in himself over the past few days (which straddled the days of his absence from the sessions, and to which he made no conscious reference)—had been a 'work station' he had been building at home. After months of indecision, he had finally got round to creating his own office space. Now that he had achieved this, he felt resentful at the thought of leaving it all behind to set up a new home with his partner. He then detailed how he had sourced all the materials for the workstation, designed it himself and created what he tellingly described as 'something out of nothing'. He was very pleased with the result. His closest friend had called round when he was 'in the thick of it', and he had felt irritated by this interruption, but his friend had in fact made 'a small observation' that he now realized had 'some relevance' to the design he had in mind. His friend was 'understated', which he liked. He sometimes wished he could be like that, but he feared that unless he imposed himself on others, as he recognized that he often did, he was at risk of being 'taken over'.

I was aware of the transferential implications of what he had been saying. I felt powerfully that he needed to impress on me that he had created his safe work enclave as an alternative to his analysis (and to the prospect of cohabiting with his partner) and that this is where he needed to retreat to—a 'station' no less, conjuring up in my mind the image of a superior, more substantial structure than our analytic workspace. Significantly he had built it himself by himself and for himself—a space from which he could control the object/me, not least through cancelling his sessions.

I was mindful too that Mr C had also seemingly lied about his reason for cancelling his sessions, since he had been evidently well enough to build his workstation. Lying was a feature in many of his relationships, a strategy he used to titrate closeness. I was aware also of another communication: of a 'nothing' state of mind that he had got into, which as I knew by now captured Mr C's experience of feeling lost, 'without spine', as he had put it on other occasions, and the meticulous care that had gone into the creation of a work station—a 'something-out-of-nothing'—that held him together in his mind.

I felt I needed to approach this defence carefully, respecting the construction whilst not ignoring the plight of its architect. In other words, I considered that I needed to intervene, but I did not think that a here-and-now transference interpretation would help. On the contrary, at this juncture, I thought that a transference interpretation would simply play into a rather predictable dynamic: I would impose on him the demand to work with me and build something together and he would simply pull away insisting that he did not need my help and that he could do the work of *analysis much better by himself. In other words, the transference interpretation might harm him in relation to the work that I was trying to do with him, namely, to help him to develop a mind of his own. I am using the word 'harm' here in a loose sense in so far as I do not believe that I would have caused serious irreparable injury to his mind, but I would have nevertheless undermined the purpose of what we were trying to do together. This is a form of 'harm' in so far as the intervention works against the patient's best interests in that moment.*

If I took up the meaning of the missed sessions this would have been 'correct' in one sense—his not coming was significant and the way he related to me now in the session was yet another instance of how he kept me 'on a leash' in his mind. But I doubt any of this would have helped him: it felt like it would have simply read as my 'long list' of things he had to attend to. Responding in this way would have been driven more by my need to do what I thought I <u>should</u> do—work in the transference—and thus I would be prioritizing my needs and transference to what 'working in the transference' connects me with in terms of my internal 'analytic object'.

At the same time not intervening did not feel appropriate either. This is a common dilemma for the therapist: silence can be helpful, and often necessary, but it can also abandon the patient who needs to be accompanied, not led. So, not intervening might be an instance of me harming the patient through omission.

So, what was in his best interests? Here I was guided by Mr C's account of how his friend had in fact 'made a small observation' that he now realized had 'some relevance' to the design of his workstation. I took this as an indication that he could take something in from his object even though he could only do so if he felt in control and superior (after all he refers to the friend's observation as 'small' and it is only granted 'some relevance' to his grander design, so he is not giving the friend that much credit, but he does at least acknowledge him). I felt that I needed to find a way to communicate that I was present, and that I could make a small contribution rather than riding in with my interpretations, thereby supporting the development of his autonomy.

Informed by my internal processing of the transference, I made a simple, descriptive observation aimed at capturing Mr C's state of mind when building his work station (i.e. the concentrated solo effort to build a safe refuge without any help from the other) and which I felt was also live in the here-and-now: "You carefully built this workstation for yourself, by yourself, from scratch, and you feel better and safer in the space it gives you". My aim was simply to begin to engage with Mr C's 'something-out-of-nothing' experience and its function in his psychic economy with as little saturation as possible so that it was consistent with supporting his capacity to discover his own mind.

Mr C replied, irritated, that of <u>course</u> (his emphasis) he had built it from scratch because he preferred to do things himself, that not even money could buy 'quality' these days. I immediately felt the brunt of his contempt as my carefully chosen words appeared to intrude into his safe enclave, imposing on him the demand to acknowledge my presence, which he had immediately to quash.

And yet in the long silence that ensued I sensed that Mr C was perhaps beginning to work with me. When he resumed speaking, he told me about a nightmare he'd had a few days earlier in which his favourite nanny (who had looked after him for many years when he was a child) was singing to him a 'simple yet soothing lullaby'. In the dream he desperately wanted to sleep, but something inside him—'like a sore tooth pulsating in anger' —had kept him awake. His thoughts were incoherent in the dream, and he feared he was going mad. He woke up in a sweat reaching out for his partner, only to realize she was not there. He then said that sometimes he worried that his procrastination might lead his partner to leave him. She was a good woman, but there were times when she was indistinguishable in his mind from his mother, and then he felt trapped. He recognized that sometimes he longed for her presence, felt he needed her, but if she was there, he could just as easily find himself wishing her away, recoiling from her embrace. This pattern tormented him as he could not see a way out.

I did not say anything although there was a great deal that could have been said, but I did not think there was any need to intervene because Mr C now appeared to be representing, through his recounting of the nightmare, and hence processing, his assault on me/his objects and on his own mind. At a not-yet-conscious level I thought that he recognized my 'simple yet soothing' attempt to reach him, just like the nanny in the dream, and how in response he had bitten me with his angry tooth. Having attacked me he was left on his own. Importantly, this biting him also disturbed

*him: he knew this was the path to a kind of madness and that it left him be-
reft of the comfort of the other (as he wakes from his nightmare, he reaches
out for his partner, but she is not there, which I also took to be a reference to
the other side of his experience of the missed sessions: he knows he needs
the analysis, but he has deprived himself of what he needs).*

*There was the risk that by not intervening at this stage I would be experi-
enced by him as not being there when he reached out and thus potentially
undermine the development of his autonomy given that psychoanalytically speaking, we are working to a notion of relational autonomy such
that we are not seeking to discourage the reality of dependency and the
need for help from the other. In the moment I was guided by the intangibles
of the live affective experience in the room, which in this instance inclined
me to trust that Mr C was able to continue without my active intervention and that my silence, in this instance, was not a withdrawal from him;
rather it was actively supportive of his autonomy.*

*Mr C paused some more and then said that his girlfriend had been upset
the previous day because they had agreed to prepare supper together,
but in the event, he had started to cook without her in order to 'surprise'
her. He observed, bemused, that this had really upset her: 'I could not understand why she was upset that I spared her the trouble of cooking! And
then she walked out in a huff, and I ended up eating alone'. He added that
she missed out on a 'jolly good meal'. At this juncture I asked a question informed by my experience in the transference of him needing the analysis to
be his own creation without any interference from me. Playing on the concrete and symbolic registers, I asked: 'Who were you cooking for?'*

*After a silence Mr C interestingly replied that my question had brought
to his mind an advertisement for meals-for-one at the local supermarket,
which he now never bought because he thought the food was full of pre-
servatives. Nowadays he was buying only organic food from a local
health food store, but this meant he could not rely on them having what
he wanted when he wanted it. He thought it was best to stick to this new
regime.*

*After another long silence he said, now in a more reflective tone, that
he could see that he had left his partner out, that he had reneged on their
agreement to cook dinner together and that she probably read into this his
inability to share his life with her, which is why she must have been upset.*

He added: 'And she's right in one way . . . just like my <u>work bench</u> [my emphasis] is for me, made by me, and no-one can interfere with this . . . I do this here all the time too . . . . If you tell me something I often feel this impulse to just tell you to shut up and my voice . . . the voice in my head as I imagine myself saying this to you sounds horrible . . . . It sounds . . . well, I can't think of how else to put it, but it's like a guttural sound, savage almost, like it's a matter of life and death.'

He then vividly relayed a story about a wildlife documentary he had seen some weeks previously where they had showed, 'in slow-frame motion', how a crocodile had 'set upon' a buffalo drinking by the water's edge. It had bitten right into him. Mr C said that he had found himself strangely very affected by this scene because it was such a calm, beautiful 'everyday scene'—the buffalo 'only taking what he needed to survive'—which was then defaced by the brutality of the attack.

Mr C then became tearful. I felt very moved by the road Mr C had travelled on in the session and the intersection of thoughts he had reached. I was struck by two details that marked, in my view, how his state of mind had progressively evolved towards a more depressive level of functioning without much active intervention from me. First, his grand 'work station', which at the beginning of the session was felt to be safer and superior to the work space of his analysis, is now referred to as a more modest 'work bench'. Second, Mr C mentions the wildlife scene that evidently moved him and is shown 'in slow-frame motion'—a detail which I took to refer to how he was now able to replay and watch, in slow motion (i.e. attentively), the scene of his own attack: how at some level he recognized that he defaced everyday exchanges, with me in the analysis, and importantly with his partner whom he feared would leave him because of this.

At this point I thought the timing was ripe for a transference interpretation because Mr C had elaborated sufficiently in his own way his experience without much interference from me: all the pieces were there for us to share an 'aerial view' (see Chapter 4) of what he was struggling with. And yet I also had to challenge myself and ask why I would make this interpretation given how the session had evolved. Why not, instead, let him know I am following him and let him continue to work over the meaning of what is forming in his own mind? I thus only said: 'You are both the crocodile and the buffalo'.

Mr C replied that he was not sure what I meant—why was he both? He could see how he was the crocodile towards others, 'biting the hand that feeds me'. He said: 'I can be aggressive to others especially when I feel under threat . . . if they try to tell me what to do . . . but no . . . this is not just about that . . . it is something about the 'hand that feeds me' . . . like not accepting your help, not letting you in'. Mr C went on in this vein for a few minutes and then said, '. . . but I cannot understand how I can be the buffalo . . . I'm intrigued . . . all I can see is his face lowered into the water bank and he is drinking peacefully . . . I am never peaceful'.

Now I thought that Mr C was actively inviting me to 'cook together': he needed my help, and I took this as a cue for intervening in a more fulsome manner: 'You have a clear view in your mind from the river looking out at the unsuspecting buffalo, who is doing the most ordinary thing: he drinks the water he needs to survive when he is set upon. I think that you recognize how you set upon the very people you need because you fear they will take you over: so you come here to your analysis with your prepared meal-for-one on which you have been feeding yourself since we met last week'.

Mr C was silent at first and then went on to say that he was aware that we had not discussed the missed sessions and that he was surprised I had not raised this as he had 'expected' me to. He now felt guilty about having missed them because he had not, in fact, been unwell: he had simply not wanted to come as he was so wrapped up in building and did not want to abandon this. He could now see that he had retreated into his DIY as a way of avoiding having to think about what sharing space with his partner brought up for him. He then said, with sadness in his voice, 'I guess I am not good at cooking with someone'.

Mr C's state of mind was now palpably mournful, but also desolate and I considered that he needed my very active presence to stay with this experience, so I took this as a further cue to intervene: 'What seems so painful is that you know meals-for-one are not good for you, that simple things may have their value, but you cannot provide them for yourself by yourself— you have to rely on others. So, in a way you are also the victim of your own bite: you are the buffalo who is set upon by a part of your mind that warns you against the dangers of allowing yourself to long for what you need in order to survive emotionally, and prevents you from taking comfort from 'everyday' moments, like working together here with me or cooking with your partner.'

I will not go further into this session. I share this excerpt because it is, in one sense, a rather mundane one in so far as the transferential implications are clear at the start of the session. It is also not unrepresentative as there are many intersections in an analytic session, just as in this one, when we could take something up in the transference directly. I can appreciate that this could have been a way of proceeding with this patient in the session. But what this excerpt also illustrates, I hope, is that the patient was able to arrive at an important and moving insight without the transference interpretation being made, but through four other interventions. Over their course the patient gradually represented his experience through recounting the nightmare and then through a series of associations that led him to the moving and harrowing scene of the crocodile and the buffalo.

The first type of intervention, I refer to as 'active-in-passive', and the other three interventions are explicitly 'active' in the sense that despite their relative under-saturation they nevertheless 'interfere' with the patient's own process because they explicitly present the therapist's mind to the patient's attention. The 'active-in-passive' intervention—which is the one I especially want to draw attention to—is the internal formulation in the therapist's mind (i.e. the analytic and ethical 'work') that informs the decision *not* to make a fulsome transference interpretation. This is then followed by the more active interventions in the form of transference-informed observations ('*You carefully built this work station for yourself, by yourself, from scratch, and you feel better and safer in the space it gives you*' and later '*You are both the crocodile and the buffalo*') and of a transference-informed question ('*Who were you cooking for?*'). All these interventions support the aim of drawing the patient's attention obliquely to the object relationship dominant in his mind in relation to his partner and to me in the transference. This way the path is laid for the patient to arrive at his own interpretation when he realizes *emotionally* that he 'cooks-for-one' in his life, including in the session, and is led to the scene of the crime against his objects and himself in the form of the attack on the buffalo by the crocodile.

Of course, not all patients have Mr C's capacity, but the point here is only to illustrate that there are varied ways of 'using' the analytic relationship that do not involve the direct interpretation of the transference. I am not suggesting that this way of working will be of equal help to all patients, but I am suggesting that ethical practice rests on our willingness to question why we do what we do in relation to whether this benefits or harms the patient. Not interpreting (Bonaminio, 1993, 2008; Gabbard, 1989) or intervening in the kind of pedestrian way I described in Chapter 4 are much underrated analytic techniques that aid the analytic process and support the development of 'a mind of one's own' and hence support the development and exercise of the patient's autonomy. In other words, considering the potential value to the patient of a transference interpretation is an ethical task as much as it is a technical question.

Both Winnicott (1969) and Bion (1976), each in their distinctive ways, have brought to our attention the importance of facilitating the patient's discovery of himself, noting how easy it is to interfere with this. Interference with the process of helping the patient to develop a mind of his own, as I suggested in Chapter 3, represents an ethical failure. Interpretations can be too saturated with the therapist's need to know. Indeed, Bion evocatively referred to the way the analyst's interventions can become 'space stoppers . . . putting an end to curiosity' (1976: 22). In a similar vein, Winnicott wisely observed:

> It is only in recent years that I have become able to wait and wait for the natural evolution of the transference arising out of the patient's growing trust in the psychoanalytic technique and setting, and to avoid breaking up this natural process by making interpretations. It will be noticed that I am talking about the making of interpretations and not about interpretations as such. It appalls me to think how much deep change I have prevented or delayed . . . by my personal need to interpret. (Winnicott, 1969: 711)

As I mentioned in Chapter 4, Bion's (1962) notion of K as a 'getting to know' (Ogden, 2004) reminds us that this challenging process can readily mobilize an internal imperative to know *the* answer. At its best an interpretation should be an expression of a K relationship with the patient to support the patient's capacity to experience and know himself as someone who has a mind.

If, as I have suggested, a fundamental aim of therapy is to help the patient to develop a mind of his own in order to support relational autonomy, then psychoanalytically beneficent interventions are in the service of stimulating the patient's own curiosity about his mind and that of others. This process supports the internalization of a capacity to reflect on his own experience—this is, ethically speaking, the psychoanalytic 'good' that I have suggested we should strive to protect. The ever-present risk in our work is that we may overextend ourselves in the direction of speculation and interpret because this is what we think we should be doing rather than interpret because the patient will be helped by it (beneficence). This represents an instance of 'interpreting-in-minus-K' where 'being a proper analyst' takes precedence in the therapist's mind over listening to the patient.

A variety of interventions can support the aim of 'illuminating a K relationship'. Asking the patient a question that deepens an exploration of a feeling or a phantasy or the associative linkages in a dream (Boesky, 1989; Sousa et al., 2003) may also engage the patient in a process of knowing about his mind as effectively as a transference interpretation. I am suggesting therefore that technique should be informed by this ethical aim (beneficence), that is the helpfulness of the interpretation of transference (and of any intervention we make) needs to be evaluated against the criterion of whether it helps stimulate the patient's capacity to represent his own subjective experience if we consider this to be one of the psychoanalytic 'goods'. For example, we need to repeatedly evaluate the extent to which the unconscious phantasies that are active in the patient's mind can be explored in a more emotionally 'persuasive' way by a here-and-now transference focus as opposed to a focus on what is happening in the patient's relationships outside the therapy room. With some patients, for example those who have few actual relationships, the transference relationship becomes a primary entry point into the patient's affective experience and into his imaginative life. For others, however, their report of current relationships outside of therapy may be affectively charged and provide sufficient immediacy for us to be able to engage the patient in a live exploration of what troubles him in his mind. Always bringing everything back to the here-and-now transference may not 'add' anything, but how we determine when this applies or not can only be guided by our understanding of the transference.

I have focused here on the interpretation of transference as an example of an intervention because it is a personal interest and to illuminate the relevance of ethics to our daily work. We could equally apply these ideas and the questions they promote to many other interventions such as the management of therapy boundaries. For example, when is our decision to not return a patient's call outside of work hours taken in the patient's best interests however upsetting it might feel for the patient (i.e. it is an instantiation of an ethical principle), and when might it instead reflect a harmful enactment of an unmetallized anger towards the patient? A primary task for us is to create and safeguard the conditions in which the patient's curiosity about his mind can flourish and to examine how our interventions support or inhibit this aim. This 'safeguarding' function emphasizes the importance of monitoring our personal equation so as to minimize impingements on the patient's space.

8
Developing the *Ethical Chóros*

*Do you observe, Meno, that I am not teaching the boy any-
thing, but only asking him questions?*

—(Socrates)[1]

As we approach the end of this book, you may consider that what
I have been advocating throughout is sensible, even uncontentious,
and yet locating ethics at the heart of our discipline is a challenging
task. It is all too easy to dilute the real demand that the call to ethics
places on us. Rules and codes of conduct cannot protect against the
unconscious pulls that we are all susceptible to. In a discussion about
the relative merits of professional codes of ethics, Levin underlines
how

> . . . the code provides a safety barrier in which attention to the work of
> self-monitoring and self-restraint can to some extent be externalized
> and automated in order to free up energy for experimental thought. We
> can more easily afford to take mental leaps when the 'real' boundaries
> and danger zones are explicitly marked. But . . . the risk of the code is
> that it becomes idealized to the point of reification, generating a cul-
> ture based on rules at the expense of reflection and freedom of thought.
> (2010: 76)

---

[1] Available at: http://www.log24.com/philo/MENOexcerpt.html.

If psychoanalysis wants to be fit for purpose in the twenty-first century, we must take a critical look at what we mean by acting ethically and how we can best support the development of this capacity in our psychoanalytic trainings. It is vital to assess whether our current trainings are conceptually and normatively well equipped to provide simultaneously ethical guidance to clinicians while providing protection to individual patients. If we train candidates according to an exclusively rule-based code of ethics or we simply schedule a few obligatory seminars on ethics, we misapprehend the ethical situation of psychoanalysis. Ethical matters in psychoanalysis—as in life more generally—cannot be fixed and solved according to set rules or focusing on a few salient ethical topics. As Levinas' philosophy brings home to us, acting responsibly towards our patients makes an ethical demand on us that at some level we will resist and at times may even fully reject. We can aspire to the ideal of timely and deeply moving interpretations that we read in published case histories where the narrative is about the transformative power of understanding and containing the patient. But there will be moments during a therapy when what the patients asks of us, and what we have in fact promised, is just too much. I would venture as far as to suggest that if we don't ever feel this, we are probably not doing psychoanalytic work.

Availing oneself totally to another person, be that our patient, or our child, or our partner, and expecting nothing in return, is a demand that far exceeds what any of us can provide without some push back, some of the time. As I have been suggesting throughout, unless we recognize the nature of this demand, we are more at risk of ethical breaches. The challenge for training is then how we can support ethical practice and encourage openness to learning from our mistakes without this becoming a persecutory experience. In this concluding chapter, I therefore outline an approach that can aid the development of the *ethical chóros* during training and beyond. In a book dedicated to ethics, I cannot ignore the important question of the ethics of teaching, hence I will also briefly touch on this, but I cannot do justice to this vast area in the context of this chapter.

Fear and shame: The enemies of learning

During my career, I undertook two separate psychoanalytic trainings—first as a psychoanalytic psychotherapist and then as a psychoanalyst.[2] These were privileged learning opportunities. I could write at length about their respective merits and how invaluable they have been to me. I share this personal detail to contextualize my upcoming criticism. In neither of these trainings was ethics discussed in a systematic and integrated manner except through a handful of seminars on confidentiality and sexual boundary violations. This remains the case in many curricula and reflects how ethics has not yet secured the place it deserves in our psychoanalytic trainings. By now you will no doubt anticipate what is coming: I believe that we would enhance our standing as a profession and support the development of better equipped therapists to deal with the inevitably of our errors and ethical breaches (conceived here broadly) and with ethical conflicts, if we could create dedicated spaces within training and beyond to consider the role of ethics. We must prioritize building up the therapist's 'ethical muscle' (Abramovitch, 2007: 449).

I began this book inviting you to 'live and love the questions' that ethics urges us to engage with. This committed curiosity is the backbone of the *ethical chóros*, but curiosity is hard-won. To be curious we need to recognize that we are missing epistemic goods, such that we can then be curious about them: I cannot be curious about something that I believe I already know. Curiosity requires an acknowledgement of insufficiency in the self (or within a specific professional group) and recognition of the need for the other who can help us with what we lack. This is why being a learner is an emotionally complex position. This is not simply connected to the transference we all have to any range of psychoanalytic ideas and their proponents, as discussed earlier. It is also about the painful aspects inherent in learning itself, that is the way any learning involves simultaneously taking something in and making it one's own (i.e.

---

[2] The first involved a training to work with patients at an intensity of three-times weekly sessions and the second involved working with patients in five-times weekly sessions.

identifying with it) whilst acknowledging the dependency on those who teach us (Lemma, 2012). The resulting sense of 'implied incompleteness and inadequacy of the self' (Rustin, 2001: 208) must be borne. It exposes us to our ignorance and the shame this can potentially mobilize. As learners, we are inevitably in the sway of our superego, a more-or-less benign internal structure.

Fear and shame are the enemies of all learning and of ethical practice. As Archangelo aptly put it: '. . . Education is about the shattering confrontation between who we are and who we are supposed to become' (2007: 335), and he might have just as easily been writing about the demands we have to manage when we focus on our ethics. If we are trainers in the field, we have a responsibility for creating training cultures that model the essence of the *ethical chóros*, avoiding the pitfalls of superego moralism. This means that the more senior we become, it is more important to share our work openly, to reveal our errors, so that we can make it possible for more junior colleagues to feel comfortable exposing their own. All too often, scientific meetings and publications conspire to create the opposite atmosphere, as we are presented with polished interpretations and the benefits of post hoc insights. At such meetings we may welcome (or perhaps at times simply tolerate) that a colleague would have approached the work differently and might therefore view our interventions as less helpful than what they might have done, but this is quite different to sitting in front of colleagues and saying: "I got this wrong, this is why I think I got it wrong, and I was not able to help this patient". Owning up to mistakes may sound virtuous but it's not always so. I am as suspicious of a *mea culpa* approach to ethics as I am of someone who cannot recognize, let alone own, their mistakes. We cannot ignore how apparent openness to our imperfections and the willingness to expose these, as Kravis shrewdly observes, on deeper analysis might not distinguish us very much at all from those whose approach to their work betrays their omniscience,

> . . . both groups are possibly defending against narcissistic injury and shame in ways that may eventuate in chronic, sequestered feelings of falseness and imposture. (Kravis, 2013: 97–98)

So, whichever position we take, we must be wary of the idiosyncratic ways in which we manage narcissistic injury and shame. It is difficult to reveal oneself to be wrong or to not know something we think we ought to know. We are all grappling with the same challenges, the shame that our flawed nature can evoke, but we each metabolize and express this differently.

A crucial part of analytic training is to help candidates to reflect on the demands made on the therapist by the very specific nature of our work (Schafer, 1994) and how this, in turn, may impact on how we relate to and use ideas and techniques. Our need for an organizing structure when we are confronted with the patient's pain may help us understand the fierce attachment we can develop to our models and preferred techniques—our so-called 'idols of the cave' (see Introduction). At its best, teaching helps candidates to approach critically and creatively the ideas with which they are presented instead of using teaching to 'facilitate the integration of generations into the logic of the present system and bring about conformity to it' (Shaull, 1996: 16). Over my professional lifetime as a psychoanalytic candidate and then as a trainer, I have observed progress in this respect. However, we need only take a cursory look at a number of curricula to note how their content shapes what is considered to be 'psychoanalysis', or what constitutes 'normal' development, for example, through what they omit to teach as much as through what they emphasize. In the past, the way we have taught, or at times altogether failed to address, the vexed question of homosexuality in our trainings is a case in point.

As educators, we all have our prejudices and passions, which is why it is important repeatedly to revisit what we teach and how we teach it. Analytic education is made all the more complicated by the fact that training to become a therapist rests on a substantive personal, experiential component, which inevitably fosters strong attachments and emotional reactions to teachers, and the content of what is studied. The primary learning context is the relational field of our personal analysis/therapy alongside the important direct experience of working with training patients under supervision.

Appropriately so, emphasis is placed during training on 'learning through experience' in these two contexts.

From the vantage point of the clinical situation too great a focus on teaching theory may be used defensively to create in the therapist the illusion of 'knowing', which may foster a premature closure of receptivity to the elaboration of unconscious experience in the analytic situation. A clinical training can, however, all too readily veer towards an under-emphasis on conceptual formulation, that is insufficient attention is devoted to supporting the process of critically thinking about why we do what we do in the consulting room and how this relates to our model of therapeutic action and the best interests of the patient. Space during training to consider these questions is essential so that candidates can elaborate their own ethical position in relation to their work. When we are teaching, it is as easy to err in the direction of oversaturation with theory as it is to leave the candidate floundering without any framework to lend meaningful form to her clinical observations and experiences, or to encourage an 'anything goes' stance that masquerades as 'integration', but that on closer scrutiny betrays a muddled way of thinking lacking internal consistency. I am therefore not advocating the pursuit of conceptual formulations for their own sake, but rather as a corrective to self-serving implicit theories or theories that lack coherence.

Going beyond the ethical floor approach: A proposed curriculum and approach to teaching ethics

Existing training in ethics mostly approximates the 'ethical floor' approach with, at one end, a focus on minimal obligations and, at the other end, a near-exclusive focus on the more egregious violations. This leaves a relative void in-between. This approach to teaching ethics is not adequate for our purposes. We need a space for consideration of the more everyday errors, ethical dilemmas, and breaches such as the ones that I have discussed in previous chapters. It goes without saying that we need to address a range of core topics, but it is only through the *integration* of ethics into the very fabric of how we train that we can support the development of the *ethical chóros*. We need an ongoing, sustained engagement with the ethics of psychoanalysis as a method and of its purpose (Alpert and Steinberg, 2017; Chervet and Porte, 2011). More to the point, and as Scarfone highlights, we need to clearly formulate the place of ethics in our training curricula to ensure that we are not only addressing the 'manifest, *professional* outer shell, which may or may not reflect the inner *personal* ethical core of the practitioner' (2017: 393).

Both Jane Kite (2016) and Sarah Ackerman (2020) have made important contributions to how we think about ethics in psychoanalysis. I share their overall sentiments and their emphasis on the need to carefully consider each case on its merits. For example, Ackerman states that 'We may even need to reinvent the rules with each patient every time we meet' (2020: 573). However, during training, guidance to 'reinvent the rules' with each patient may be too abstract to be of practical use. I have no doubt that this was not Ackerman's intention, but the case-by-case approach that informs her advice invites some qualification. Each case undoubtedly requires attention to the specifics (you will recall the importance of 'specification'—see Chapters 2 and 7) but these specifics are helpfully considered against the conceptual pillars of a principled approach. Particularity does not negate the value of universal principles that must be applied in specific ways. The latter provide a second layer of scrutiny that encourage us to consider the ethical dilemma or intervention from a range of angles that, in turn, brings into vision salient ethical considerations that we might otherwise neglect.

No doubt, the suggestions I will shortly share for how to teach ethics will not suit everybody's preferences. As I mentioned in the 'Introduction', my own approach to this area has been informed by the time I have spent over the years studying psychotherapy manuals, writing a psychotherapy manual (Lemma et al., 2011), and working on psychotherapy competence frameworks. The level of specification such activities require can be used in a reductionistic manner, but it need not lead to such a desultory use. At their best, operationalizing terms and outlining models are forms of applied systematic thinking that have in-built check points. This helps us to question our terms, frames of reference, our beliefs, and, most importantly, ourselves. This is the essence of applied ethics.

I want to make a strong case for sustained and integrated teaching on ethics throughout training and post qualification. We have rightly argued for the importance of integrating teaching on diversity into our curricula and for this to *not* be a standalone unit. Ethics also deserves to be integrated into how we teach so that we expand the range of the questions we can explore and critically debate as we consider psychoanalytic ideas, technique, and the very nature of psychoanalytic knowledge and power relations. What we select to teach ought to be at least in part examined from the standpoint of questions such as: 'How does this help our candidates do the best for their patients?' Or 'How does it protect the patient from potential harms?' Or 'How does how we teach ensure accessibility of the analytic model to a broader, more inclusive range of patients?' This is not a matter of thinking that 'it would be good to do so, if only we had time'. It is essential. This is not because we exist in a world of increasing governance, regulation, and litigation and therefore we need to be on top of these matters—although all this is true. It is essential because the ethical integrity of our practice is fundamental to our work. Therefore, we need to have reflective spaces and conceptual frameworks that help us to safeguard the best that psychoanalytic therapy and psychoanalysis have to offer to further our patients' best interests.

We cannot ignore, as Kravis (2013) highlights in his discussion of why we hate our work, that my emphasis in this book on the necessity to acknowledge the need for *ongoing* ethical monitoring of ourselves in relation to our work, no matter how senior we are, or how humble we think we are, may sit uncomfortably. In practice, as Kravis points out, any reminder that we are blind to some aspects of what drives our work even when we consciously acknowledge this risk, means that '... healthy pride will have to attach itself primarily to becoming skilled at accepting one's perpetual need for self-scrutiny', without sinking into the disheartened feeling that the predication of wisdom and expertise eludes those who are most honest about their flaws

(Kravis, 2013: 92). This is easier said than done. Anticipating our natural resistance to keep going back to ourselves, Freud advocated regular reimmersion in analysis at different stages of our careers:

> Every analyst should periodically—at intervals of five years or so—submit himself to analysis once more, without feeling ashamed of taking this step. This would mean, then, that not only the therapeutic analysis of patients' but his own analysis would change from a terminable into an interminable task. (1937: 249)

The ideas I will share next may simply not be helpful, or deemed necessary, and I welcome debate on this. However, even if you are persuaded that my emphasis on ethics is justified, we must be wary of reifying this into an 'ethical ideal'. As Ackerman notes, we can only aspire to be more ethical. If this becomes all too concrete in our minds, we are more at risk of acting unethically:

> . . . This ideal is necessary as a commitment to doing what is best for the patient but holding the tension of knowing that we inevitably fall short of this ideal is itself a vital part of doing what is best for the patient. (2020: 563)

How to embed teaching in applied ethics: A personal view

When I decided to write this book, I committed myself to not retreating away in the lofty tower of abstract ideas and ideals and instead take the risk of spelling out the practical training implications of the arguments I set out in earlier chapters.[3] As a thought experiment, I asked myself what I would do if I had carte blanche and I was offered the opportunity to (re)design a psychoanalytic therapy or psychoanalysis curriculum with regards to teaching ethics. I am

---

[3] Other useful papers that outline how the authors approach teaching ethics to psychoanalytic candidates are by Abramovitch (2007) and Molofsky (2014).

passionate about the importance of integrating ethics into our curricula, but my passion does not make me right. I am sure there are different ways of addressing the problem, and the approach I will now outline is not intended to be the 'right' one. However, I hope that by sharing some concrete ideas, it will offer a springboard for thinking about what and how to teach that can then be discussed and adapted for the purposes of different trainings. What follows is where I have got to in my thinking.

Given that once we embark on a training, we relatively quickly start to see patients, my view is that as candidates we should be exposed at the outset to thinking about ethics, that is thinking about what it is that we are offering our patients (i.e. what is the purpose of the analytic encounter?), considering the ethical risks inherent to our role and our method and questioning the nature of our responsibility. As trainers, our role is to reveal to candidates how ethics helps us to think about how we can offer psychoanalytic help in a way that benefits the patient, does not harm the patient, is fair, truthful, and supports his autonomy. This is where we should begin our training, not only with teaching about Freud or Klein.

As I set out in Chapter 3, ethics begins with an articulation of what we think we are doing when we agree to take on a patient. Of course, our capacity to articulate the conceptualization of our work and its instantiation will be refined many times over through clinical experience and through exposure to the theories that will help us to frame this experience. However, before we see the first patient, we really ought to have given at least some thought to what we are aiming to do, have fleshed out some of the controversies about how we understand the purpose of psychoanalytic interventions, and hence how we establish the conditions for meaningful consent to the therapy, and have considered in what way ethics lies at the core of our work. We can begin to address this in an extended workshop-type format early on in training, facilitated by preferably two workshop leaders who don't share the same approach to psychoanalysis and who can help the group to reflect on these important questions. I suggest the facilitation by seminar leaders from different theoretical orientations because it is only through exploring differences that we create a space for thinking from which individual positions can then be elaborated. As I was studying ethics, I was often struck by how the live ethical debates that I attended, and the ones I had to participate in, sometimes arguing for positions at variance with my own presumptions, provided a fertile space for thinking through the live experience of observing 'difference in action'.

I suggest that the first workshop, preferably run towards the end of the first term and spanning two sessions, should be framed around the question: 'What is the purpose of psychoanalysis/psychotherapy? Two good papers to start off the discussion are Thomas Ogden's (2019) 'Ontological psychoanalysis or "What Do You Want to Be When You Grow Up?"' and Jonathan Lear's (2009) 'Technique and final cause in psychoanalysis: Four ways of looking at one moment'. The workshops I have in mind would be very applied, and would aim to help candidates to develop a meta position about how they understand the purpose of what it is they think they are doing when they practice psychoanalysis and its varied, less intensive therapeutic applications such as brief therapy or group therapy. Some of the helpful questions that can be explored in smaller group exercises might include reflection on the difference between 'what we say' and 'what we do' and between 'what we claim' and 'what we truly aim for'. As we embark on our clinical journeys with our patients, we would all benefit from some frank conversations about these matters. This sets the tone for a training culture that nurtures individuality and frames psychoanalytic knowledge as provisional. This cultural 'tone' is supported when seminar leaders are prepared to expose their differences. In the workshops I am sketching out, it would be important to create a space for each of the seminar leaders to give a succinct (say five minutes) presentation of the bare bones of how they would describe what they do and how they believe it could help the patient. This provides some material for discussion and debate.

This two-sessions workshop can then be followed with applied ethics seminars, which ideally benefit from retaining a workshop type format with small-group exercises alongside teaching and discussion. To this end, I will share a proposed curriculum with suggested readings that I found particularly helpful as I immersed myself in this literature. Although the proposed seminars are intended to cover theoretical questions, the delivery of the seminars should ensure there is an applied focus to give candidates the opportunity to apply ethical thinking to real-life clinical dilemmas and to the way they practice. The aim is to create opportunities to exercise the ethical muscle that sustains good practice. Specific ethical dilemmas arise all the time and we could never address all eventualities in a comprehensive manner during training. Moreover, I don't believe this to be necessary or the best way to teach ethics. The priority is to develop the skill of approaching these scenarios more systematically. This can be achieved through group exercises inviting candidates to think through different ethical dilemmas and provide justification of their decision. Faced with a patient who, for example, unexpectedly loses his job and cannot pay for his sessions, but is clearly very distressed and needs help, and a therapist who is herself struggling financially and cannot afford to lose a fee, metapsychology alone or primarily, or an understanding of the transference, are not going to provide a comprehensive enough context for thinking through the ethical questions that will allow the therapist to find a way to manage such conflicting interests. In the end, our decisions are not only clinical decisions. They are also moral decisions. Processing a few such scenarios in small groups provides opportunities for candidates to use the five principles to think through how they arrive at a decision about how to act.

The meaning we give to our work and the reasons we have for our actions with our patients are relevant issues for ethical consideration because they already contain a normative evaluation of the situation. Normative knowledge embodied in practice can be made explicit by ethical analysis. Especially useful during the seminars are case examples that explore those clinical scenarios, as Abramovitch advocates, where the therapist's choice could not be straightforwardly conceptualized as choosing, as he puts it '. . . between good and bad, but between bad and worse—the so-called 'grey areas' between what is clearly forbidden and what is absolutely allowed' (2007: 450).[4]

---

[4] The American Psychoanalytic Association (APsaA) ethics casebook provides a good source of examples (Dewald and Clark, 2007).

Another important focus would be how we think about the very notion of a 'boundary', such as how do we define it and how do we know when we have crossed it?[5] It will be down to the seminar leader to weave such questions into the discussion and to select applied examples throughout the ten seminars.

Ideally the ten seminars would benefit from being complemented by *ethics masterclasses* scheduled later in the training when candidates have been working with patients for some time. These would offer the opportunity to think about some thorny ethical dilemmas or treatment failures with the benefit of senior clinicians willing to share some of their difficult ethical decisions and/or errors. Presentations by senior colleagues could alternate with a masterclass where one of the candidates is invited to do the same, with a more senior colleague chairing the masterclass and teasing out the salient ethical challenges, guiding the group through thinking about the ethical principles that are at stake and most likely in tension with each other.

The first goal of the masterclasses would be therefore to develop the experience of applying ethical principles to the case being presented with the aim of building competence in applied ethical analysis relevant to psychoanalytic practice. The masterclasses should strive to balance discussion of clinical dilemmas that illustrate the challenge of balancing competing ethical principles with consideration of individual sessions or whole therapies that have not had a good outcome. This would address the second goal of the masterclasses: to contribute to consolidating a training culture that can accommodate the reality of failure and help candidates to reach out

---

[5] As Levin observes in his discussion of the notion of a 'boundary':

It may be . . . that the term also reflects our wishful thinking. We would all like to believe that the interpersonal aspects of psychoanalysis can be refereed objectively, as in a tennis match, where the ball lands either on or inside the line, or outside it, most of the time. But the boundaries we allude to, though real enough, stubbornly resist definition; they waver, like the frame, with circumstances and personalities, precisely because they are part of a liminal process . . . everything depends upon context and contingent details. No fantasy of a fixed and precise boundary or rule will truly protect analyst or analysand from the psychic risks of exploring unconscious mental life. (Levin, 2010: 74)

for help rather than conceal struggles because they feel this would reflect poorly on them.

Maintaining ethical fitness post-qualification

During training we are in the privileged position of receiving a lot of supervision. This ensures more protection for both therapist and patient. The evidence we have garnered over the years with regards to sexual boundary violations suggests that such transgressions are more likely *post* training and the more senior we get. So, more experience can breed more omnipotence at the very point when we are less supervised and is more likely to result in unethical behaviour:

> The recurrence of the construct of the 'third' reminds us that the analytic setting involves a radical privacy between two people, a fertile field for mutual self-deception that may go unchecked. While analytic training occurs in the context of triad—patient, analytic candidate, and supervising analyst—the third party often disappears after graduation. As I have long advocated, restoring a 'third' by using a consultant early in a difficult analytic process may be our best hope to prevent traumatic betrayals . . . . Even though consultation can be subverted by leaving out key developments in the analysis, it also offers the opportunity to transform the dyad into a triad in which the analyst carries an internalized 'third' into each session with the patient. (Gabbard, 2015: 583)

It is essential, therefore, to consider how we can support each other post-qualification to maintain an ethical focus. My proposal is that as part of the annual process of professional registration, Continuing Professional Development (CPD) obligations could specify a requirement to undertake one extended clinical-ethics consultation once a year with a senior colleague focusing on a case where something has gone wrong. This would not only ensure that we support awareness of errors but also that we have dedicated and required spaces where we can safely explore such experiences with an explicit focus on the ethics of our work. More to the point, by embedding this in our CPD requirements, it normalizes in the profession that we *expect* such errors and that monitoring these is part of our responsibility no matter how experienced we are.

Inevitably there is the risk that if we were to institute such a requirement as part of the renewal of registration, this may encourage 'confession' of very minor errors in a mechanistic manner instead of encouraging genuine reflection on the difficult aspects of our work.[6] There is no full proof way to regulate this, but we can increase the chances of this becoming a meaningful process of reflection if we commit to creating training cultures that place ethics at their core. Moreover, the purpose of the consultation would include, where necessary, challenging a colleague if it looked like they were engaging in a tick-box exercise rather than being receptive to thinking critically about their work. My suggestion is intended to embed a focus on ethics at the heart of how we monitor our work. However, such a requirement, if it were formalized, would only be helpful if these consultations were genuinely safe spaces to explore the ethics of practice, no different to supervision (which we do make a compulsory requirement of registration) except for their specific focus. And a final thought: if training institutions really want to get behind the focus on ethics and change training cultures, they could also sponsor a prize for a paper on a treatment failure as a contribution to the learning of that institution.

The ethics of pedagogy: Keep asking the questions

So far, I have considered the ethics of the therapist but not of those amongst us who also take up a training function. As educators we have a captive audience. This affords power, and hence responsibility. What is it to be ethical as a psychoanalytic educator? Both Socrates and Freud agreed that teaching was an 'impossible profession'. For Freud this was so along with 'government and

---

[6] I am grateful to Heather Wood for drawing my attention to this risk.

psychoanalysis' (Freud, 1937: 248). If teaching is an impossible profession, how should we understand and carry out our task? What are our obligations?

I cannot hope to answer these complex and fundamental questions in any exhaustive manner here. Suffice it to say that we have obligations to our students as individual subjects who entrust us with their desire to learn. But we are also training them to offer a psychological intervention that can benefit and harm people, so we have a further responsibility towards the public. As educators, we are inevitably implicated in the drama of ethical production and its failures. Since, as educators, we are instrumental in the development of candidates, and because of our institutional roles we are 'producers' of subjects and society, we must examine the profound and consequential responsibility this entails.

There will be inevitably, and there should be, critical questioning of the suggestions I have made in this chapter. Some of the possible objections will be practical ones because of the implications that flow from my proposals, not least that whenever we suggest more seminars on one topic, this inevitably means cutting back on others. Anyone who is involved in training will recognize this perennial challenge. This fact, in and of itself, exposes that at the heart of education lie normative considerations that are seldom systematically examined as such. For example, a decision to devote, say, ten seminars to Freud and three to ethics reflects the normative commitments embedded in our conceptualization of what matters in forming a psychoanalytic therapist, that is of the kind of therapist we want to fashion. So, an important ethical question we are confronted with is this: when we apportion seminars to the various topics, in what way are ten seminars on Freud going to better serve the interests of the patient who is ultimately one of the prime beneficiaries of all this learning? How do these seminars contribute to minimizing the potential harm to the patient that he may be exposed to during an analytic process relative, say, to seminars on ethics, or diversity, or whatever else you want to throw in the mix? There is, of course, no right answer to these questions, but the ethics of education require us to grapple with them.

Ethics, as we have seen, should not be reduced to a tick-box exercise in the form of codes. Teaching ethics ideally strives to support an engagement with ethics in the ancient sense of the pursuit of the right way to proceed in our relationship with others—our patients—and the ongoing struggle this demands. Supplanted by imperatives of liability management and morality, the ethical conditions of relating are all too readily side-lined. In our teaching, the priority is to protect the emphasis on the latter. Part of our responsibility as educators is to consider how the subject—be it the patient, the therapist, the seminar leader— is given in discourse to be figured or thought. In other words, being an ethical educator involves thinking about the forms of thought that we impart to candidates as an ethical matter. To make this idea more practical, it means that as a seminar leader, or as the organizer of a curriculum, we concern ourselves with what thoughts our teaching makes possible or impossible and with what other disciplines we need to draw on to ensure that more expansive thought is possible. We need to consider, too, what should be our ethical response to external events that challenge our and our students' identities, beliefs, and relationships. Global pandemics, discrimination, wars, the rise of digital media usage, climate change—to name but a few of the realities and changes that we are all witnessing on a global scale—all need to be thought about in relation to how we teach, what we teach, and how this positions us ethically towards each other as colleagues and towards the patients our students will work with. Acting ethically as a trainer therefore involves an ongoing commitment to engage in a radical analysis of our psychic investments and our position in society (Taubman, 2010). It is the exploration of these domains and the willingness to contemporaneously question our choice(s) while making a choice(s), that constitutes an ethical position.

Finally, we cannot ignore another vital training function: ethics must go beyond the moral principles of individual ethics and pay attention to the moral life that dwells among the institutions in which we train, which inevitably reflect the dominant structures of society.[7] For example, Dimen was clear that

---

[7] This is an area I have not had the space to address in this book, but it is integral to ethical practice.

> . . . the phenomenon of sexual transgression between analyst and pa-
> tient is insufficiently addressed as long as it is deemed to be exclusively
> psychological. Since it is also a social matter . . . it means to be under-
> stood by means of social as well as psychological concepts. And since it
> is a group matter, it must be addressed by the group of which it is a pro-
> perty. (2021: 29)

There is an urgent need to describe more clearly the institutional and environmental contexts that mediate moral action. This is vital to the reform that our psychoanalytic institutions need with respect to questions of power and diversity of various kinds. Those of us who take on training roles share a similar responsibility namely, to create learning cultures that are open to scrutiny and engaged with disciplines that can bring new perspectives to our own discipline. Developing a capacity to be critical (i.e. questioning) of psychoanalysis and of our individual practice is essential to our survival and development as a discipline. Because we work increasingly in an external context of complaints, risk of liability, and threat of legal action against us, discussion about ethical matters can all too quickly give way to a focus on how we protect ourselves from such risks rather than focusing on how we protect our patients. It behoves us to ensure that we create spaces where ethical matters can be reflected on non-defensively, giving due consideration to how as individual practitioners and as a discipline we can create value *and* contribute to harm and use these reflections to identify where change is needed.

Ten seminars curriculum outline

Seminar 1 The therapist's ethical responsibility

In this seminar candidates are invited to explore the nature of psychoanalytic responsibility—what is the therapist responsible for—through consideration of the different kinds of asymmetries that are inherent to a patient-therapist relationship and given the therapist's inevitable subjectivity. It also introduces two key ideas: (1) therapist error and fallibility as a constant backdrop to our practice rather than as something that happens infrequently and (2) the inevitable conflict of interests between the patient's needs and desires and the therapist's.

Suggested reading:

Kite, J. (2016). The fundamental ethical ambiguity of the analyst as person. *Journal of the American Psychoanalytic Association*, 64(6): 1153–1171.

Renik, O. (1993a). Analytic interaction: conceptualizing technique in light of the analyst's irreducible subjectivity. *The Psychoanalytic Quarterly*, 62: 553–571.

Nacht, S. (1962). The curative factors in psychoanalysis. *International Journal of Psychoanalysis*, 43: 206–211.

Slochower, J. (2003). The analyst's secret delinquencies. *Psychoanalytic Dialogues*, 13(4): 451–469.

Seminar 2 The ethics of working through in the countertransference

This seminar traces the evolution of the concept of countertransference from Freud's original understanding right through to contemporary conceptualizations with a specific focus on the *ethical implications* of these conceptual shifts. The aim is to invite candidates to critically reflect on the relative merits and risks of 'too narrow' or 'too broad' an understanding of countertransference and to engage with the contributions of the intersubjective school of psychoanalysis.

Suggested reading:

Hinshelwood, R. (2012). On being objective about the subjective: Clinical aspects of intersubjectivity in contemporary psychoanalysis. *International Forum of Psychoanalysis*, 21(3–4): 136–145.

Pick, I. B. (1985) Working through in the countertransference. *International Journal of Psychoanalysis* 66: 157–166.

Racker, H. (1957). The meanings and uses of countertransference. *The Psychoanalytic Quarterly*, 26: 303–357.

Wilson, M. (2013). Desire and responsibility: The ethics of countertransference experience. *The Psychoanalytic Quarterly*, 82(2): 435–476.

Seminar 3   On loving and hating our work

In this seminar, the focus is squarely placed on creating an open thinking space about how our work can be rewarding and emotionally demanding and about how non-recognition of our loving, sexual, and hateful feelings towards the patient represent potential ethical tipping points.

Suggested reading:

Kravis, N. (2013). The analyst's hatred of analysis. *The Psychoanalytic Quarterly* 82: 89–114.

Moss, D. (2013). An addendum to Kravitz: An appreciative note on hating one's work. *The Psychoanalytic Quarterly*, 82: 115–124.

Winnicott, D. W. (1949). Hate in the countertransference. *International Journal of Psychoanalysis*, 30: 69–74.

Seminar 4   An ethics for psychoanalysis

This seminar provides an opportunity to introduce candidates to the bioethical principled approach and to consider its relevance to psychoanalytic practice, including consideration of how we can approach the question of consent to a psychoanalytic intervention. This seminar would benefit from some applied examples to provide the candidates with an opportunity to test out the value of such an approach to psychoanalytic work.

Suggested reading:

Beauchamp, T. (2003). Methods and principles in biomedical ethics. *Journal of Medical Ethics*, 29(5): 269–274.

Brenner, A. and Cather, C. (2015). Using a "virtues" approach to ethical challenges in psychoanalytic psychotherapy. In: *The Oxford Handbook of Psychiatric Ethics* (Vol. 1). Oxford: Oxford University Press

Ackerman, S. (2020). Impossible ethics. *Journal of the American Psychoanalytic Association*, 68(4): 561–582.

Kirshner, L. (2012). Toward an ethics of psychoanalysis. *Journal of the American Psychoanalytic Association*, 60(6): 1223–1242.

Scarfone, D. (2017). On "That Is Not Psychoanalysis": Ethics as the main tool for psychoanalytic knowledge and discussion. *Psychoanalytic Dialogues*, 27: 392–400.

Wilson, M. (2012). The flourishing analyst, responsibility, and psychoanalytic ethics. *Journal of the American Psychoanalytic Association*, 60(6): 1251–1258.

Seminar 5   The inevitability of our values and their impact on psychoanalytic work

In this seminar the focus is on facilitating a free-flowing discussion about the part played by our values in theory building and in practice and on the relevance of the patient's values. Consideration is also given to whether psychoanalytic work can or should be concerned with morality.

Suggested reading:

Black, D. (2020). The working of values in ethics and religion. *International Journal of Psychoanalysis*, 101(5): 992–1013.

Groarke, S. (2018). Moral experience and the unconscious. *Philosophy, Psychiatry & Psychology*, 25(2): 137–142.

Harcourt, E. (2018a). Psychoanalysis, the good life, and human development. *Philosophy, Psychiatry & Psychology*, 25(2): 143–147.

Harcourt, E. (2018b). Madness, badness, and immaturity: Some conceptual issues in psychoanalysis and psychotherapy. *Philosophy, Psychiatry & Psychology*, 25(2): 123–136.

Meissner, W. W. (1994). Psychoanalysis and ethics: Beyond the pleasure principle. *Contemporary Psychoanalysis*, 30: 453–472.

Seminar 6   Confidentiality and writing about our patients

This seminar focuses on the ethics of publication, inviting candidates to reflect on whether it can ever be justifiable to publish without full consent and if the decision *is* to publish, to consider the extent to which it affects the analytic process and how this might be mitigated sufficiently to justify publication. Questions of consent, of the timing of such requests to the patient, and consideration of the merits of alternative ways to disseminate knowledge without publishing case material, are some of the key questions that would benefit from being covered.

Suggested reading:

Ackerman, S. (2018). (How) can we write about our patients? *Journal of the American Psychoanalytic Association*, 66(1): 59–81.

Aron, L. (2016). Ethical considerations in psychoanalytic writing revisited. *Psychoanalytic Perspectives*, 13(3): 267–290.

Lear, J. (2003). Confidentiality as a virtue. In: C. Levin, A. Furlong, and M. K. O'Neil (eds) *Confidentiality: Ethical Perspectives and Clinical Dilemmas*. New York: Routledge, pp. 3–18.

Tuckett, D. (2000). Reporting clinical events in the journal: Towards the construction of a special case. *International Journal of Psychoanalysis*, 81: 1065–1069.

Report of the IPA Confidentiality Committee (2018). https://www.ipa.world/IPA_DOCS/Report%20of%20the%20IPA%20Confidentiality%20Committee%20(English).pdf.

Seminar 7   Sexual boundary violations

Without question, therapists frequently have sexual and romantic feelings and fantasies about their patients. This seminar will promote discussion about the erotic transference and countertransference, and consider the devastating impact of sexual boundary violations, aiming to tease out how we understand the very notion of a 'boundary', giving due consideration to the ethical notions of bodily integrity and bodily autonomy.

Suggested reading:

Celenza, A. (2010). The analyst's need and desire. *Psychoanalytic Dialogues*, 20(1): 60–69.

Saketopoulou, A. (2021). Does the sexual have anything to do with sexual boundary violations? In: C. Levin (ed.) *Social Aspects of Sexual Boundary Trouble in Psychoanalysis: Responses to the Work of Muriel Dimen*. London: Routledge, pp. 101–128.

Gabbard, G. (2017). Sexual boundary violations in psychoanalysis: A 30-year retrospective. *Psychoanalytic Psychology*, 34(2): 151–156.

Dimen, M. (2011). Lapsus linguae, or a slip of the tongue? *Contemporary Psychoanalysis*, 47(1): 35–79.

Dimen, M. (2017). Eight topics: A conversation on sexual boundary violations between Charles Amrhein and Muriel Dimen. *Psychoanalytic Psychology*, 34(2): 169–174.

Seminar 8   The ethical risks of online therapy

This seminar will focus on the risks and benefits of virtual relating and of the virtual setting for psychotherapy with specific attention devoted to the impact of virtual space on self-governance. Consideration is given to the ethical risks introduced by the remote setting and of our quotidian interface with different types of media, using the example of Patient-Targeted Googling as a point for discussion and application of bioethical principles.

Suggested reading:

Clinton, B., Silverman, B., and Brendel, D. (2010). Patient-Targeted Googling: The ethics of searching online for patient information. *Harvard Review of Psychiatry*, 18(2): 103–112.

Lemma, A. (2017) *The Digital Age on the Couch*. London: Routledge. Chapters 4 and 5.

Suler, J. (2004). The online disinhibition effect. *Cyberpsychology & Behavior*, 7(3): 321–326.

Seminar 9   Psychoanalytic failures and why apologizing matters

In this seminar candidates are invited to reflect on the nature of a psychoanalytic treatment failure, on how they might discuss an 'error' with a patient and consider the intrapsychic and interpersonal functions of an apology in order to examine the practical implementation of the Duty of Candour.

Suggested reading:

Benjamin, J. (2009). A relational psychoanalysis perspective on the necessity of acknowledging failure in order to restore the facilitating and containing features of the intersubjective relationship (the shared third). *The International Journal of Psychoanalysis*, 90: 441–450.

Celenza, A. (2017). Lessons on or about the couch. *Psychoanalytic Psychology*, 34(2): 157–162.

Elise, D. (2015). Unravelling: Betrayal and the loss of goodness in the analytic relationship. *Psychoanalytic Dialogues*, 25: 557–571.

Kächele, H. and Schachter, J. (2014). on side effects, destructive processes, and negative outcomes in psychoanalytic therapies: Why is it difficult for psychoanalysts to acknowledge and address treatment failures? *Contemporary Psychoanalysis*, 50(1–2): 233–258.

Seminar 10   Silence, gossip, and guilt: Institutional challenges to change

This closing seminar focuses on individual and institutional responsibilities when we are confronted with knowledge that a colleague has transgressed with a patient. Candidates will be encouraged to examine the issue of collective silence and the ensuing private 'gossip' in the face of ethical breaches and how this is enabling, and implicates us all, to varying degrees, in sustaining a culture of narcissism within training institutions and organizations.

Suggested reading:

Burka, J., Sowa, A., Baer, B. A., Brandes, C. E., Gallup, J., Karp-Lewis, S., Leavitt, J., and Rosbrow, P. (2019). From the talking cure to a disease of silence: Effects of ethical violations in a psychoanalytic institute. *International Journal of Psychoanalysis*, 100: 247–271.

Gabbard, G. (2016). The group as complicit in boundary violations: Commentary on Dimen. *Journal of the American Psychoanalytic Association*, 64: 375–380.

Gentile, K. (2018). Assembling justice: Reviving nonhuman subjectivities to examine institutional betrayal around sexual misconduct. *Journal of the American Psychoanalytic Association*, 66: 647–678.

Grossmark, C. (2017). Candidates' responses to sexual boundary violations. *Psychoanalytic Dialogues*, 27(1): 79–88.

Levin, C. (2021). Introduction: Social preconditions of psycho-sexual violations in psychoanalysis: Reflections on the ethics of Muriel Dimen. In: C. Levin (ed.) *Social Aspects of Sexual Boundary Trouble in Psychoanalysis: Responses to the Work of Muriel Dimen*. London: Routledge.

Sandler, A. and Godley, W. (2004). Institutional responses to boundary violations: The case of Masud Khan. *International Journal of Psychoanalysis*, 85(Pt 1): 27–44.

Slochower, J. (2017). Don't tell anyone. *Psychoanalytic Psychology*, 34: 195–200.

Epilogue: A Plea for a Measure of Irony

'No genuinely human life is possible without irony', believed Kierkegaard (1989: 326) because, for him, irony paves the way for an ethical life with the attendant responsibility.[1] I began the book sharing with you one of my favourite poets. I want to conclude now with another favourite: this time it is a book about irony by the philosopher and psychoanalyst, Jonathan Lear (2011). In his Kierkegaardian treatise of irony (with a psychoanalytic twist), what Lear means by irony is not the gap between what one is and what one claims or aspires to be. Rather, he means the calling into question of the entire framework of assumptions, aspirations, and ideals that go with a specific social identity, be that of being a 'teacher' or a 'psychoanalyst'. The experience of irony, as Lear understands it, disrupts our sense of who we are, alerting us to the shifting sands of identity that lurk beneath the surface of apparent unity and certainty. We might say, then, that irony is the call to make the implicit explicit so that our assumptions and personal investments can be examined. This involves reckoning with our unpalatable vulnerability and fallibility, which nevertheless contains the seeds of redemption from the impoverishment of an unexamined life:

> ... the concepts with which we understand ourselves and live our lives have a certain vulnerability built into them. Ironic existence thus has a claim to be a human excellence because it is a form of truthfulness. It is also a form of self-knowledge: a practical acknowledgment of the kind of knowing that is available to creatures like us. (Lear, 2011: 31)

Lear suggests that irony manifests as a distinctive mode of questioning that plays a positive role in ethical life (see also Thornton, 2022). At its core, applied ethics, as I have presented it in this book, is the instantiation of an ironic approach to our work in so far as it calls into question the very foundations of who we are, of what we do, and what we believe in. A focus on ethics is a way of signing up to the importance of being self-reflexive and self-reflective, considering our own methods and theoretical approaches as open questions that benefit from being revisited over time and from different angles. As Bacon (1889) cautioned, our 'idols of the cave' can imprison us and may prevent us from stepping outside of our world as we know it and value it, to see something differently.

When we bring together applied ethics and psychoanalysis, we have access to two immeasurably rich frameworks that can support an ironic approach to our clinical

---

[1] Kierkegaard clearly distinguishes between romantic irony and Socratic irony. I am using the term in its Socratic sense, which is associated with the elenctic method, that is questioning the (colloquial) knowledge and beliefs of the interlocutor.

work, to our teaching and to our everyday lives. Ethical practice requires an ongoing commitment to disrupting our most deeply rooted identities—the central pillars of normative orientation in our journeys of becoming. Being ironic about our work involves engaging our curiosity about whether our practices and our codes of ethics have become no more than worn clichés that prop up our professional identity but on closer examination have been denuded of their ethical dimension. It takes courage to revisit our assumptions and ways of doing psychoanalytic therapy or psychoanalysis and to ask ourselves, for example, why do I make *this* interpretation and not another and do so in a way that truly prioritizes the patient's best interests?

As therapists and as trainers of therapists, we hold a central position in the knowledge economy. This requires us to appreciate the importance of epistemic goods and the relations of power inherent in their development and exchange. The analytic setting, as much as the training setting, are not simply places of treatment or professional learning respectively. They are also lived experiences in which subjects such as 'the patient' and 'the psychoanalytic therapist' are being formed within often implicit relations of power. Striving to be an ethical therapist is to be compelled at every step to think about what we are doing, why we are doing it, and how we are doing it. We need all the help we can get to stay on course and get better at identifying ethical tipping points. Theories and conceptual models are always at risk of converting the inevitable uncertainty that we all face in our work with patients into an illusory sense that we can predict and know. I hope that the principles examined in this book will not be used in this manner. This would only turn the therapist and patient as ethical subjects into generalized notions of 'a therapist' and of 'a patient' losing all the specificity of the unique dynamic that belongs to that analytic dyad and only to that dyad. That said, I also hope that I have managed to convey the added value of using a principled ethical framework, and its merits for us all, not least when we are candidates and are striving to develop the mental architecture to support the *ethical chóros* in our minds.

Writing this book has been personally challenging. It is impossible to write about this subject without taking a close, uncomfortable look at oneself. I like to think that I have done my best for the patients who have sought my help. That is precisely where part of the challenge lies: it can only be 'my' best. We must bear the guilt that comes with knowing that at times we have not helped the patient as much as he needed to be helped. We must bear knowing that this is not always because the patient could not be helped by psychotherapy alone, or didn't want to be helped, but because *we* specifically could not help due to our personal limitations or the limitations of our method, or of the setting in which the therapy unfolds,[2] or a combination of all these factors. As we revisit such situations, it is prudent to be mindful of the seductions of the 'benefit of hindsight' state of mind. This can become a narcissistic indulgence if all we do is deploy our psychoanalytic theories in a self-serving manner to make 'what went wrong' fall neatly into place in our minds so as to not

---

[2] For example, for some patients an intensive psychoanalysis might be viable in the context of a residential therapeutic community setting where there are adjunct supportive structures, but not in the context of a private therapy setting.

unduly disturb our beliefs and allegiances, and we don't learn from the experience and change how we work going forwards.

Questioning ourselves keeps us on the ethical track. This is easier said than done, which is why we need spaces during training and beyond where we can be supported to exercise the kind of discipline and self-scrutiny that allows our work to thrive. Personal therapy and supervision are invaluable to this process but, in my view, insufficient for the task. Ours is indeed an 'impossible profession'. It is as unique in the demands it places on us as it is in its rich returns. Throughout my professional experiences working in different mental health settings, and specifically offering psychoanalytic help, I have never once wished I was doing something else. Studying ethics and the process of writing this book have nevertheless confronted me with how easy it is at times to slip into 'pretending' to be a psychoanalytic therapist or psychoanalyst. By 'pretending' I do not mean that we play-act the role but rather that we unselfconsciously operate in a rote manner and are then at risk of serving our interests before the patient's. We can only begin to grapple with our ethics when we catch ourselves pretending in this manner and commit ourselves to questioning how this could be so.

Glossary

Applied ethics also called practical ethics or moral philosophy—is a branch of philosophy. It examines and defines principles for moral behaviour and applies them to real world scenarios. In contrast to traditional ethical theory—concerned with purely theoretical problems such as, for example, the development of a general criterion of goodness—applied ethics takes its point of departure in practical ethical challenges and attempts to answer the question of how people should act in specific situations, but without needing to find agreement on which moral theory to apply. This is because the method of applied ethics rests on a systematic analysis of the facts at hand and the related harms and benefits of a specific situation. It balances or prioritizes different values and interests.

Bioethics is the study of moral issues pertaining to the fields of medical treatment, clinical research, and overall patient care. It aims to establish what health professionals and researchers should and should not do. In the 1970s bioethics was not yet established as a field, though there was increasing recognition that this was needed, not least because of the ethical questions raised in the 'Nuremberg Code' (1949),[1] 'The Declaration of Helsinki' (1964),[2] and 'The Belmont Report' (1976),[3] which all proposed guidelines for human research and argued that scientists and healthcare practitioners have moral obligations to uphold.

Deontology is a normative theory originally associated with Immanuel Kant who believed that it's wrong to treat people as mere instruments to meet our own goals, without respecting them as people. Kantians argue that you should treat all people with dignity and act only on rules that everyone can endorse. Deontologists are thus concerned with rules and obligations and propose that a moral act stems from a sense of duty. An act can be the right thing to do even if it produces a bad consequence, that is duty should be performed for its own sake (this is also known as Kant's 'categorical imperative'), even when obedience of the rule (e.g. we must never lie) does not create the best outcome.

---

[1] The Nuremberg Code, "Trials of War Criminals before the Nuremberg Military Tribunals under Control Council Law No. 10", Vol. 2, pp. 181–182. Washington, DC: US Government Printing Office, (1949).

[2] Declaration of Helsinki: Recommendations Guiding Doctors in Clinical Research, 18th World Medical Assembly, Helsinki, Finland (June 1964).

[3] The Belmont Report: Ethical Principles and Guidelines for the Protection of Human Subjects of Research, National Commission for the Protection of Human Subjects of Biomedical and Behavioral Research. (18 April 1979).

Duties

> *Prima facie* duties are those that we ought to perform, in and of themselves, and must be fulfilled unless in conflict with an equal or stronger duty.
>
> *Actual* duties require examining the respective weights of competing prima facie duties.

Epistemic injustice refers to a wrong done to someone as a knower or transmitter of knowledge such that due to unjustified prejudice, someone is unfairly judged to not have the knowledge or reasonable beliefs that they actually have. The theory was first proposed by Miranda Fricker (2007), according to whom there are two forms of epistemic injustice:

> *Testimonial injustice* occurs when the level of credibility attributed to a speaker's word is reduced by prejudice operative in the hearer's judgement and not because the testimony itself is unreasonable. These prejudices can be related to race, gender, accent, age, and others and impact people in many areas of life: economic, educational, professional, sexual, legal, political, religious, and more.
>
> *Hermeneutical injustice* results when testimonial injustice is so persistent and socially patterned (as anything driven by prejudice is likely to be), that it contributes to hermeneutical marginalization. Hermeneutical injustice then is about cases where the individual lacks the concepts to adequately understand or communicate an experience.

Ethical chóros, derived from the Greek, χῶρος meaning a clearly defined space/environment—a dwelling space (which is quite different from a 'chorus' (χορός), a band of singers and dancers, even though it is phonetically similar). This is a term I am introducing for the first time to denote a *principled internal space* in the therapist's mind that regulates clinical practice through supporting self-questioning in relation to the work with the patient and the obligations we have towards him, the most fundamental of which is that we must create and safeguard in our mind a dwelling space for the patient and his singularity. It is a part of the therapist's internal setting whose primary function is to monitor the tensions arising from the confrontation with the therapist's responsibility for the patient, the emotional demands that ensue, and the defences this can mobilize in the therapist so as to minimize ethical breaches and clinical errors.

Ethics of care, first developed by the psychologist Carol Gilligan, is a feminist philosophical perspective that uses a relational and context-bound approach toward morality and decision making. This approach developed from a study conducted in the 1970's on how girls look at ethics. Gilligan found that in relation to boys, the moral development of girls tended to come from compassion instead of being justice-based. From this study, Gilligan proposed that ethics should be focused on relationships instead of emphasizing autonomy and rules. Her theory challenges traditional moral theories as male-centric and problematic to the extent they omit or downplay values and virtues usually culturally associated with women or with roles that are often cast as 'feminine', such as prioritizing our feelings and the relationships we share.

Ethical theory is a general explanation, rooted in specific principles, of when and why actions are wrong or not. The four main theories are deontology, utilitarianism, virtue ethics, and care ethics.

Principlism was articulated by Tom Beauchamp and James Childress, first in 1977, as an approach to ethical decision making. They developed a set of principles that most ethicists could agree to, arguing that these core principles (beneficence, non-maleficence, respect for autonomy, and justice) are detailed enough to guide analyses and decisions, yet flexible enough to adapt to different cases and cultures.

Prudential value refers to the 'good' for a specific person. A prudent act is one that will generally help make one's life go better and, as such, enhances well-being.

Utilitarianism is the most prominent version of *consequentialism*. It is associated with the ideas of Jeremy Bentham and John Stuart Mill. It subscribes to a view that the morality of an action depends on its consequences, that these consequences matter with respect to whether they increase or decrease happiness (or avoid the 'most bad'), and that happiness is the happiness of everyone who might be associated with the action concerned, not just the person who performs it. At its most basic, the theory states that something is moral, or good, when it produces the greatest amount of good for the greatest number of people. Utilitarians typically argue that we are obligated to do whatever action has the best *overall* consequences for all who are affected by the action.

Virtue ethics is a normative theory rooted in the ideas of Plato and Aristotle. It defines good actions as ones that embody virtuous character traits, like courage, loyalty, or wisdom. As an approach to ethics, it emphasizes the virtues, or moral character, in contrast to an emphasis on duties or rules (deontology) or on the consequences of actions (utilitarianism). According to some virtue ethicists, an action is right if, and only if, it is what a virtuous person would characteristically do under the circumstances. Virtue ethicists argue that actions must help people form better characters or live better lives.

Well-being refers to what is intrinsically (or non-instrumentally) good for someone. Whereas instrumental goods like wealth are valuable only as a means to something else, well-being is what ultimately makes someone's life go well. There are three main theories of well-being:

Desire satisfaction theories propose that the fulfilment of a person's desires is what makes their life go well. Importantly, it is not the feeling or experience of a desire being satisfied that matters, but that a desire is in fact satisfied.

Hedonism considers well-being to be rooted in an overall positive balance of pleasure over pain (both broadly construed). In other words, our lives go best when they have the greatest amount of pleasure.

Objective list theories claim there can be things that make a person's life go better which are neither pleasurable nor desired by them, such as friendship, knowledge, virtuous behaviour, and health. Such items are 'objective' in the sense of being concerned with facts beyond both a person's conscious experience and/or their desires.

References

Abramovitch, H. (2007). Stimulating ethical awareness during training. *Journal of Analytical Psychology*, 52: 449–461.

Ackerman, S. (2018). (How) can we write about our patients? *Journal of the American Psychoanalytic Association*, 66(1): 59–81.

Ackerman, S. (2020). Impossible ethics. *Journal of the American Psychoanalytic Association*, 68(4): 561–582.

Akhtar, S. (2002). Forgiveness: Origins, dynamics, psychopathology, and technical relevance. *Psychoanalytic Quarterly*, 71: 175–212.

Akhtar, S. (2018). Humility. *The American Journal of Psychoanalysis*, 78(1): 1–27.

Allen, J. (2008). Psychotherapy: The artful use of science. *Smith College Studies in Social Work*, 78(2–3): 159–187.

Alpert, J. and Steinberg, A. (2017). Introduction: Sexual boundary violations: A century of violations and a time to analyze. *Psychoanalytic Psychology*, 34(2): 144–150.

Appel, J. (2011). Toward a psychodynamic approach to bioethics. *American Journal of Psychoanalysis*, 71: 58–66.

Archangelo, A. (2007). A psychoanalytic approach to education. *Psychoanalysis, Culture & Society*, 12: 332–348.

Aristotle (1953). *Nicomachean Ethics*. Harmondsworth: Penguin.

Aron, L. (2016). Ethical considerations in psychoanalytic writing revisited. *Psychoanalytic Perspectives*, 13(3): 267–290.

Ashley, F. and Ells, C. (2018). In favor of covering ethically important cosmetic surgeries: Facial feminization surgery for transgender people. *The American Journal of Bioethics*, 18(12): 23–25.

Atterton, P. (2007). The talking cure: The ethics of psychoanalysis. *The Psychoanalytic Review*, 94(4): 553–576.

Austin. J. L. (1975). *How to Do Things with Words*. J. O. Urmson and M. Sbisà. (eds) (2nd edn). Oxford: Clarendon Press.

Bacon, F. (1889). *Novum Organum*. T. Fowler (ed.) (2nd edn). Oxford: Clarendon Press.

Barratt, B. (2015). Boundaries and intimacies: Ethics and the (re)performance of 'The Law' in psychoanalysis. *International Forum of Psychoanalysis*, 24(4): 204–215.

Batson, C., Kobrynowicz, D., Dinnerstein, J., Kampf, H., and Wilson, A. (1997). In a very different voice: Unmasking moral hypocrisy. *Journal of Personality and Social Psychology*, 72: 1335–1348.

Bauman, Z. (1993). *Postmodern Ethics*. Chichester: Wiley.

Beauchamp, T. (2003). Methods and principles in biomedical ethics. *Journal of Medical Ethics*, 29(5): 269–274.

Beauchamp, T. and Childress, J. (2013). *Principles of Biomedical Ethics*. Oxford: Oxford University Press.

Beckett, S. (1983). *Worstword Ho!* New York: Grove Press.

Bell, D. (2011). Knowledge as fact and knowledge as experience: Freud's constructions in analysis. *Bulletin of the British Psychoanalytical Society*, 47(1): 9–21.

Benjamin, J. (1998). *Shadow of the Other: Intersubjectivity and Gender in Psychoanalysis*. New York: Routledge.

Benjamin, J. (2004). Beyond doer and done to: An intersubjective view of thirdness. *Psychoanalysis Quarterly*, 73(1): 5–46.

Benjamin, J. (2006). Two-way streets: Recognition of difference and the intersubjective third. *Differences (Bloomington, Ind.)*, 17(1): 116–146.

Benjamin, J. (2009). A relational psychoanalysis perspective on the necessity of acknowledging failure in order to restore the facilitating and containing features of the intersubjective relationship (the shared third). *International Journal of Psychoanalysis*, 90: 441–450.

Bion, W. R. (1962). *Learning from Experience*. London: Heinemann.

Bion, W. R. (1963). *Elements of Psycho-Analysis*, 4: 14–16 (downloaded from Pep-Web). London: Routledge.

Bion, W. (1976). *Four Discussions with W. R. Bion*. Scotland: Clunie Press.

Bion, W. (Ed.). (1978). *Four discussions with W. R. Bion*. London: Clunie Press.

Black, D. (2020). The working of values in ethics and religion. *International Journal of Psychoanalysis*, 101(5): 992–1013.

Black, D. (2021). Dante, duality, and the function of allegory. *Raritan*, 41(1): 19–164.

Blass. R. (2003). On ethical issues at the foundation of the debate over the goals of psychoanalysis. *International Journal of Psychoanalysis*, 84(4): 929–943.

Boesky, D. (1989). The questions and curiosity of the psychoanalyst. *Journal of the American Psychoanalytical Association*, 37: 579–603.

Bolognini, S. (2005). Il bar nel deserto. Simmetria e asimmetria nel trattamento di adolescenti. *Rivista Psicoanal*, 51: 33–44.

Bonaminio, V. (1993). Del non interpretare: Alcuni spunti per una rivisitazione del contribuito di M. Balint e due frammenti clinici. *Rivista di Psicoanalisi*, 39: 453–477.

Bonaminio, V. (2008). The person of the analyst: Interpreting, not interpreting, and countertransference. *The Psychoanalytic Quarterly*, 77: 1105–1146.

Borys, D. and Pope, K. S. (1989). Dual relationships between therapist and client: A national study of psychologists, psychiatrists, and social workers. *Professional Psychology, Research and Practice*, 20(5): 283–293.

Boulanger, G. (2012). Psychoanalytic witnessing. *Psychoanalytic Psychology*, 29(3): 318–324.

Bovens, L. (2008). Apologies. *Proceedings of the Aristotelian Society*, 108: 219–239.

Braithwaite, J. (1999). Restorative justice: Assessing optimistic and pessimistic accounts. *Crime and Justice*, 25: 1–127.

Brenner, A. and Cather, C. (2015). Using a "virtues" approach to ethical challenges in psychoanalytic psychotherapy. In: Sadler, John Z., K. W. M. Fulford, and Werdie (C.W.) van Staden (eds) *The Oxford Handbook of Psychiatric Ethics* (Vol. 2). Oxford: Oxford University Press, pp. 1264–1275.

Brenman-Pick, I. (1985). Working-through in the countertransference. *International Journal of Psychoanalysis*, 66: 157–166.

Britton, R. (2004). Subjectivity, objectivity, and triangular space. *The Psychoanalytic Quarterly*, LXXIII(1): 47–61.

Britton, R. and Steiner, J. (1994). Interpretation: Selected fact or overvalued idea?. *International Journal of Psychoanalysis*, 75: 1069–1078.

Burka, J., Sowa, A., Baer, B. A., Brandes, C. E., Gallup, J., Karp-Lewis, S., Leavitt, J., and Rosbrow, P. (2019). From the talking cure to a disease of silence: Effects of ethical violations in a psychoanalytic institute. *International Journal of Psychoanalysis*, 100: 247–271.

Busch, F. (2010). Distinguishing psychoanalysis from psychotherapy. *International Journal of Psycho-Analysis*, 91: 23–34.

Butler, J. (2005). *Giving an Account of Oneself*. New York: Fordham University Press.

Butler, J. (2006). *Precarious Life: The Power of Mourning and Violence*. New York: Verso Books.

Butler, J. (2012). *Parting Ways*. New York: Columbia University Press.

Calef, V. and Weinschel, E. (1980). The analyst as the conscience of the analysis. *International Review of Psychoanalysis*, 7: 279–290.

Candilis, P., Gray, S., Howe, E., Gennaro, K., Nesheim, R., Sisti, D., and Van Loon, J. (2018). Psychiatric professionalism for the 21st century: The committee on professionalism and ethics, group for: The advancement of psychiatry. *Psychodynamic Psychiatry*, 46(4): 537–548.

Caper, R. (1999). *A Mind of One's Own: A Kleinian View of Self and Object*. London: Routledge.

Celenza, A. (2010). The analyst's need and desire. *Psychoanalytic Dialogues*, 20(1): 60–69.

Chamberlain, M. (2022). *Misogyny in Psychoanalysis*. Oxford: Firing the Mind.

Chervet, B. and Porte, J. (eds) (2011). *L'éthique du psychoanalyste*. Paris: Presses Universitaires de France.

Chetrit-Vatine, V. (2014). *The Ethical Seduction of the Analytic Situation: The Feminine-Maternal Origins of Responsibility for the Other*. London: Karnac/Ipa.

Clarke, J. (2019). We need to talk about Fabian: Klein's 'lost' theory of projective identification and the social construction of gender/queer objects. *Psychoanalytic Psychotherapy*, 33(3): 192–217.

Clinton, B., Silverman, B., and Brendel, D. (2010). Patient-targeted Googling: The ethics of searching online for patient information. *Harvard Review of Psychiatry*, 18(2): 103–112.

Corpt, E. (2018). The ethics of listening in psychoanalytic conversations. *Psychoanalysis, Self and Context*, 13(3): 220–228.

Crastnopol, M. (2019). The analyst's Achilles' heels: Owning and offsetting the clinical impact of our intrinsic flaws. *Contemporary Psychoanalysis*, 55(4): 399–427.

Crenshaw, K. (1991). Mapping the margins: Intersectionality, identity politics, and violence against women of color. *Stanford Law Review*, 43(6): 1241–1299.

Crisp, R. (2021). *Well-Being, The Stanford Encyclopaedia of Philosophy*. Edward N. Zalta (ed.). https://plato.stanford.edu/entries/well-being/

Cutliffe, J. and Links, P. (2008). Whose life is it anyway? An exploration of five contemporary ethical issues that pertain to the psychiatric nursing care of the person who is suicidal, part 2. *International Journal of Mental Health Nursing*, 17(4): 246–254,

De Araujo, R. and Kowacs, C. (2019). Patient-Targeted 'Googling:' When therapists search for information about their patients online. *Psychodynamic Psychiatry*, 47(1): 27–38.

Denis, P. (2008). In praise of empiricism. In: D. Tuckett et al. (eds) *Psychoanalysis Comparable and Incomparable*. London: Routledge, pp. 38–49.

Denis, P. (2011). Pour une éthique de la méthode. In: B. Chervet and J.-M. Porte (eds) *L'éthique du psychanalyste, Monographie et débats de psychanalyse*. Paris: Presses Universitaires de France, pp. 75–82.

Dewald, P. and Clark, R. (2007). *Ethics case Book of the American Psychoanalytic Association* (2nd edn). New York: American Psychoanalytic Association.

Dimen, M. (2011). Lapsus linguae, or a slip of the tongue? *Contemporary Psychoanalysis*, 47(1): 35–79.

Dimen, M. (2017). Eight topics: A conversation on sexual boundary violations between Charles Amrhein and Muriel Dimen. *Psychoanalytic Psychology*, 34(2): 169–174.

Dimen, M. (2021). Rotten apples and ambivalence: Sexual boundary violations through a psychosocial lens. In: C. Levin (ed.) *Social Aspects of Sexual Boundary Trouble in Psychoanalysis: Responses to the Work of Muriel Dimen*. London: Routledge, pp. 29–42.

Donnet, J.-P. (2011). Enjeux éthiques de la méthode analytique. In B. Chervet and J.-M. Porte (eds) *L'éthique du psychanalyste, Monographie et débats de psychanalyse*. Paris: Presses Universitaires de France, pp. 42–54.

Drozek, R. P. (2019). Psychoanalysis as an ethical process: Ethical intersubjectivity and therapeutic action. *Psychoanalytic Dialogues*, 28(5): 538–556.

Earp, B. (2014). Hymen 'restoration' in cultures of oppression: How can physicians promote individual patient welfare without becoming complicit in the perpetuation of unjust social norms? *Journal of Medical Ethics*, 40(6): 431.

Eichenberg, C. and Herzberg, P. Y. (2016). Do therapists Google their patients? A survey among psychotherapists. *Journal of Medical Internet Research*, 18(1): e3–e3.

Eissler, K. (1974). On some theoretical and technical problems regarding payment of fees for psychoanalytic treatment. *International Review of Psychoanalysis*, 1: 73–101.

Elise, D. (2015). Unravelling: Betrayal and the loss of goodness in the analytic relationship. *Psychoanalytic Dialogues*, 25: 557–571.

Ellison, N. B., Steinfield, C., and Lampe, C. (2010). Connection strategies: Social capital implications of Facebook-enabled communication practices. *New Media & Society*, 13: 873–892.

Erikson, E. (1976). Psychoanalysis and ethics—avowed and unavowed. *International Review of Psychoanalysis*, 3: 409–414.

Felman, S. (1982). Psychoanalysis and education: Teaching terminable and interminable. *Yale French Studies*, 63(63): 21–44.

Ferenczi, S. (1933). Confusion of tongues between adults and the child. *Contemporary Psychoanalysis*, 24(2): 196–206.

Ferro, A. (2009). *Mind Works*. London: Routledge.

Fletcher, G. (2016). *The Philosophy of Well-being: An Introduction*. New York: Routledge.

Fonagy, P., Luyten, P., Allison, E., and Campbell, C. (2019). *Mentalizing, Epistemic Trust and the Phenomenology of Psychotherapy*. https://discovery.ucl.ac.uk/id/eprint/10076243/1/Fonagy_Mentalizing%20and%20phenomenology_revised.pdf

Francis Inquiry. (2013). https://www.health.org.uk/about-the-francis-inquiry. Accessed on 28/01/23.

Freud, S. (1909). Letter from Sigmund Freud to C. G. Jung, June 7, 1909. The Freud/Jung Letters: The Correspondence Between Sigmund Freud and C. G. Jung 41: 230–232 (p. 231).

Freud, S. (1912a). *Recommendations to Physicians Practicing Psychoanalysis*. S.E. 12. London: Hogarth Press.

Freud, S. (1913). On *Beginning Treatment: Further Recommendations on the Technique of Psychoanalysis*. S.E. 12. London: Hogarth Press.

Freud, S. (1919). *Lines of Advance in Psychoanalytic Therapy*. S.E. 17. London: Hogarth Press.

Freud, S. (1937). *Analysis Terminable and Interminable*. S.E. 23. London: Hogarth Press.

Fricker, M. (2007). *Epistemic Injustice: Power and the Ethics of Knowing*. Oxford: Oxford University Press.

Fricker, M. (2011). Powerlessness and social interpretation. In: D. Steel and F. Guala (eds) *The Philosophy of Social Science Reader*. London, UK: Routledge, pp. 39–50.

Fricker, M. (2016). Epistemic injustice and the preservation of ignorance. In: R. Peels and M. Blaauw (eds) *The Epistemic Dimensions of Ignorance*. Cambridge: Cambridge University Press, pp. 144–159.

Frosh, S. (2011). The relational ethics of conflict and identity. *Psychoanalysis, Culture & Society*, 16(3): 225–243.

Frosh, S. (2015). Beyond recognition: The politics of encounter. *Psychoanalysis, Culture & Society*, 20(4): 379–394.

Frosh, S. and Baraitser, L. (2003). Thinking, recognition, and otherness. *The Psychoanalytic Review*, 90(6): 771–789.

Gabbard, G. (1989). On 'doing nothing' in the psychoanalytic treatment of the refractory . . . . *International Journal of Psychoanalysis*, 70: 527–534.

Gabbard, G. (2015). On knowing but not knowing in the aftermath of traumatic betrayal: Discussion of paper by Dianne Elise. *Psychoanalytic Dialogues*, 25: 579–585.

Gabbard, G. (2016). The group as complicit in boundary violations: Commentary on Dimen. *Journal of the American Psychoanalytic Association*, 64: 375–380.

Gabbard, G. (2017). Sexual boundary violations in psychoanalysis: A 30-year retrospective. *Psychoanalytic Psychology*, 34(2): 151–156.

Gentile, K. (2018). Assembling justice: Reviving nonhuman subjectivities to examine institutional betrayal around sexual misconduct. *Journal of the American Psychoanalytic Association*, 66: 647–678.

Gilligan, C. (1982). *In a Different Voice: Psychological Theory and Women's Development*. Harvard: Harvard University Press.

Gillon, R. (2003). Ethics needs principles—four can encompass the rest—and respect for autonomy should be 'first among equals'. *Journal of Medical Ethics*, 29(5): 307–312.

Gans, J., and Counselman, E. (1996). The missed session: A neglected aspect of psychodynamic psychotherapy. *Psychotherapy (Chicago, Ill.)*, 33(1): 43–50.

Glas, J. (2021). Psychoanalytic ethics, maintaining psychic reality in the intermediate space. *International Journal of Psychoanalysis*, 102(3): 479–491.

Gordon, J., Rauprich, O., and Vollmann, J. (2011). Applying the four-principle approach. *Bioethics*, 25(6): 293–300.

Groarke, S. (2018). Moral experience and the unconscious. *Philosophy, Psychiatry & Psychology*, 25(2): 137–142.

Grossmark, C. (2017). Candidates' responses to sexual boundary violations. *Psychoanalytic Dialogues*, 27(1): 79–88.

Gruenberg, P. (1995). Nonsexual exploitation of patients: An ethical perspective. *Journal of American Academy of Psychoanalysis*, 23: 425–434.

Harcourt, E. (2018). Psychoanalysis, the good life, and human development. *Philosophy, Psychiatry & Psychology*, 25(2): 143–147.

Harcourt, E. (2018). Madness, badness and immaturity: Some conceptual issues in psychoanalysis and psychotherapy. *Philosophy, Psychiatry & Psychology*, 25 (2): 123–136.

Harcourt, E. (2021). Epistemic injustice, children and mental illness. *Journal of Medical Ethics*, 47 (11), 729–735.

Harris, A. (2007). Discussion of Eyal Rozmarin's 'An other in psychoanalysis'. *Contemporary Psychoanalysis*, 43(3): 361–373.

Hegel, G. (1977). *Phenomenology of Spirit*. (A. V. Miller, trans.) Oxford, England: Oxford University Press. (Original work published 1807.)

Heimann, P. (1950). On countertransference. *International Journal of Psychoanalysis*, 31: 81–84.

Heinonen, E. and Nissen-Lie, H. (2020). The professional and personal characteristics of effective psychotherapists: A systematic review. *Psychotherapy Research*, 30(4): 417–432.

Helmreich, J. (2015). The apologetic stance. *Philosophy & Public Affairs*, 43(2): 75–108.

Henrich, J. (2020). *The WEIRDest People in the World: How the West Became Psychologically Peculiar and Particularly Prosperous*. Macmillan.

Herranz, G. (2002). The Origin of Primum Non Nocere. *British Medical Journal*, 324: 1463.

Herring, J. and Wall, J. (2017). The nature and significance of the right to bodily integrity. *Cambridge Law Journal*, 76(3): 566–588.

Higgins, J. (2020). Cognising with others in the we-mode: A defence of 'first-person plural' social cognition. *Review of Philosophy and Psychology*, 12(4): 803–824.

Honneth, A. (2005). *The Struggle for Recognition: The Moral Grammar of Social Conflicts*. Reprinted. Cambridge: Polity Press.

Hook, J. and Devereux, D. (2018). Sexual boundary violations: Victims, perpetrators and risk reduction. *BJPsych Advances*, 24(6): 374–383.

Inan, I. (2012). *The Philosophy of Curiosity*. New York: Routledge.

Jackson, H. and Nuttall, R. L. (2001). A relationship between childhood sexual abuse and professional sexual misconduct. *Professional Psychology, Research and Practice*, 32(2): 200–204.

Jacobs, T. (2001). On misreading and misleading patients: Some reflections on communications, miscommunications and countertransference enactments. *International Journal of Psychoanalysis*, 82: 653–670.

Jent, J., Eaton, C., Merrick, M., Englebert, N., Dandes, S., Chapman, A., and Hershorin, E. (2011). The Decision to Access Patient Information from a Social Media Site: What Would You Do? *Journal of Adolescent Health*, 49(4): 414–420.

Jiménez, J. (2009). Grasping psychoanalysts' practice in its own merits. *International Journal of Psychoanalysis*, 90: 231–248.

Joffe, W. and Sandler, J. (1968). Comments on the psychoanalytic psychology of adaptation, with special reference to the role of affects and the representational world. *International Journal of Psychoanalysis*, 49: 445–454.

Kächele, H. and Schachter, J. (2014). On side effects, destructive processes, and negative outcomes in psychoanalytic therapies: Why is it difficult for psychoanalysts to acknowledge and address treatment failures? *Contemporary Psychoanalysis*, 50(1-2): 233–258.

Kahane, C. (2018). Death and fallibility in the psychoanalytic encounter: Mortal gifts by Ellen Pinsky (review). *American Imago*, 75(3): 455–469.

Kierkegaard, S. (1989). *The Concept of Irony*. In: H. Hong and E. Hong (eds and trans.), Princeton, New Jersey: Princeton University Press.

Kirshner, L. (2012). Toward an ethics of psychoanalysis. *Journal of the American Psychoanalytic Association*, 60(6): 1223–1242.

Kite, J. (2016). The Fundamental Ethical Ambiguity of the Analyst as Person. *Journal of American Psychoanalysus Association*, 64(6):1153–1171.

Knapen, S., van Diemen, R., Hutsebaut, J., Fonagy, P., and Beekman, A. (2022). Defining the concept and clinical features of epistemic trust. *The Journal of Nervous and Mental Disease*, 210(4): 312–314.

Kolmes, K. and Taube, D. O. (2014). Seeking and finding our clients on the Internet: Boundary considerations in cyberspace. *Professional Psychology, Research and Practice*, 45: 3–10.

Kong, C. (2017). *Mental Capacity in Relationships: Decision-Making, Dialogue, and Autonomy*. Cambridge: Cambridge University Press.

Kravis, N. (2013). The analyst's hatred of analysis. *Psychoanalytic Quarterly*, 82: 89–114.

Kreuger, D. (Ed.) (1986). *The Last Taboo*. New York: Brunner/Mazel.

Lacan, J. (1992). *The Seminar of Jacques Lacan: Book VII The Ethics of Psychoanalysis 1959–1960*, J. Miller, (ed.); J. Forreter (trans.). New York: W.W. Norton & Co.

Lear, J. (2003). Confidentiality as a virtue. In: C. Levin, A. Furlong, and M. K. O'Neil (eds) *Confidentiality: Ethical Perspectives and Clinical Dilemmas*. New York: Routledge, pp. 3–18.

Lear, J. (2009). Technique and final cause in psychoanalysis: Four ways of looking at one moment. *International Journal of Psychoanalysis*, 90(6): 1299–1317.

Lear, J. (2011). *A Case for Irony*. Harvard, MA: Harvard University Press.

Lemma, A. (2017). *The Digital Age on the Couch: Psychoanalytic Practice and New Media*. London: Routledge.

Lemma, A., Roth, A., and Pilling, S. (2008). The Competences Required to Deliver Effective Psychoanalytic/ Psychodynamic Therapy: Clinician Version. Department of Health, publication pending, available at: www.ucl.ac.uk/CORE.

Lemma, A., Roth, A., and Pilling, S. (2009). The Competences Required To Deliver Effective Interpersonal Psychotherapy: Clinician Version. Department of Health, publication pending, available at: www.ucl.ac.uk/CORE.

Lemma, A., Target, M., and Fonagy, P. (2011). *Brief Dynamic Interpersonal Therapy: A Clinician's Guide*. Oxford: Oxford University Press.

Lemma, A. and Caparrotta, L. (eds) (2014). *Psychoanalysis in The Technoculture Era*. London: Routledge.

Lemma, A., and Savulescu, J. (2023). To be, or not to be? The role of the unconscious in transgender transitioning: Identity, autonomy, and well-being. *Journal of Medical Ethics*, 49(1): 65–72.

Lemma, A. (2010). *Under the Skin: A Psychoanalytic Study of Body Modification*. London: Routledge.

Lemma, A. (2012). Some reflections on the 'teaching attitude' and its application to teaching about the use of the transference: A British view. *British Journal of Psychotherapy*, [Online] 28(4): 454–473.

Lemma, A. (2013). Transference on the couch. In: R. Olsner (ed.) *Transference Today*. London: Routledge.

Lemma, A. (2014). The body of the analyst and the analytic setting: reflections on the embodied setting and the symbiotic transference. *International Journal of Psychoanalysis*, 95(2): 225–244.

Lemma, A. (2019). Il legame estetico: l'uso del corpo dell'analista e del corpo della stanza di analisi da parte del paziente. *Rivista di Psicoanalisi*, 65: 107–127.

Lemma, A. (2022a). *Transgender Identities*. London: Routledge.

Lemma, A. (2022b). Customising the body: From omnipotence to autonomy. In: J. Arundale (ed.) *The Omnipotent State of Mind*. London: Routledge, pp. 68–82.

Lyotard, J, (1983). *Le Differend*. Paris: Les Éditions de Minuit.

Levin, C. (2021). Introduction: social preconditions of psycho-sexual violations in psychoanalysis: Reflections on the ethics of Muriel Dimen. In: Levin, C. (ed.) *Social Aspects of Sexual Boundary Trouble in Psychoanalysis: Responses to the Work of Muriel Dimen*. London: Routledge, pp. 1–26.

Levin, C. (2010). The liminal smile: Ethics in psychoanalysis and the problem of regulation. *Canadian Journal of Psychoanalysis*, 18: 60–85.

Levinas, E. (1969). *Totality and Infinity: An Essay on Exteriority*. Pittsburgh: Duquesne University Press.

Levinas, E. (1981). *Otherwise than Being, or, Beyond Essence*. Pittsburgh: Duquesne University Press.

Levinas, E. (1985). *Ethics and Infinity. Conversations with Philippe Nemo*. Pittsburgh: Duquesne University Press.

Levinas, E. (1986). 'Dialogue with Emmanuel Levinas,' interview with Richard Kearney. In: R. Cohen (ed.) *Face to Face with Levinas*. Albany: State University of New York, pp. 13–33.

Levinas, E. (1998). *Of God Who Comes to Mind*. California: Stanford University Press.

Loewald, H. (1960). On the therapeutic action of psychoanalysis. *International Journal of Psychoanalysis*, 41: 16–33.

Løgstrup, K. (2020). *Ethical Concepts and Problems*. Oxford: OUP.

Luyten, P. and Blatt, S. (2013). Interpersonal relatedness and self-definition in normal and disrupted personality development: Retrospect and prospect. *The American Psychologist*, 68(3): 172–183.

Luyten, P., Campbell, C., and Fonagy, P. (2022). The fear of insignificance from a socio-communicative perspective: Reflections on the role of cultural changes in Carlo Strenger's thinking. *Psychoanalytic Psychology*, 39(1): 20–26.

Lyndon, A., Bonds-Raacke, J., and Cratty, A. D. (2011). College students' Facebook stalking of ex-partners. *Cyberpsychology, Behavior, and Social Networking*, 47: 711–716.

Mason, R. (2011). Two kinds of unknowing. *Hypatia*, 26(2): 294–307.

McCoy Brooks, R. (2013). The ethical dimensions of life and analytic work through a Levinasian lens. *The International Journal of Jungian Studies*, 5(1): 81–99.

Meissner, W. W. (1994). Psychoanalysis and ethics: Beyond the pleasure principle. *Contemporary Psychoanalysis*, 30: 453–472.

Merritt, A., Effron, D., and Monin, B. (2010). Moral self-licensing: When being good frees us to be bad. *Social and Personality Psychology Compass*, 4(5): 344–357.

Mill, J. S. (1910). *On Liberty*. London: J. M. Dent and Sons.

Mills, C. (2022). Undoing ethics: Butler on precarity, opacity and responsibility. In: C. Mills (ed.) *Butler and Ethics*. Edinburgh: Edinburgh University Press, pp. 41–64.

Molofsky, M. (2014). Teaching professional ethics in psychoanalytic institutes: Engaging the inner ethicist. *The Psychoanalytic Review*, 101(2): 197–217.

Monin, B. and Miller, D. (2001). Moral credentials and the expression of prejudice. *Journal of Personality and Social Psychology*, 81(1): 33–43.

Moss, D. (2013). An addendum to Kravitz: An appreciative note on hating one's work. *Psychoanalytic Quarterly*, 82: 115–124.

Nozick, R. (1969). Coecion. In: Sidney Morgenbesser, Patrick Suppes, and Morton White, (eds) *Essays in Honor of Ernest Nagel*. New York. St Martin's Press. pp. 440–472.

Nussbaum, M. (2000). *Women and Human Development: The Capabilities Approach*. Cambridge, UK: The Press Syndicate of the University of Cambridge.

Ogden, T. (1992). Comments on transference and countertransference in the initial analytic meeting. *Psychoanalytic Inquiry*, 12(2): 225–247.

Ogden, T. (1994). The analytic third: Working intersubjectively with clinical facts. *International Journal of Psychoanalysis*, 75: 3–19.

Ogden, T. (2004). An introduction to the reading of Bion. *International Journal of Psychoanalysis*, 85(2): 285–300.

Ogden, T. (2019). Ontological psychoanalysis or 'what do you want to be when you grow up?'. *The Psychoanalytic Quarterly*, 88(4): 661–684.

Omaggio, N. et al. (2018). Have you ever Googled a patient or been friended by a patient? Social media intersects the practice of genetic counseling. *Journal of Genetic Counseling [Online]*, 27(2): 481–492.

O'Neill, O. (2002). *Autonomy and Trust in Bioethics*. Cambridge: Cambridge University Press.

Oshana, M. (2014). *Personal Autonomy and Social Oppression: Philosophical Perspectives* (Vol. 65). London: Routledge.

O'Shaughnessy, E. (1999). Relating to the superego. *International Journal of Psychoanalysis*, 80(5): 861–870.

Peltz, M. and Gabbard, G. O. (2001). Speaking the unspeakable: Institutional reactions to boundary violations by training analysts. *Journal of the American Psychoanalytic Association*, 49(2): 659–673.

Pick, I. B. (1985). Working through in the countertransference. *International Journal of Psychoanalysis*, 66: 157–166.

Pilgrim, D. (2022). *Identity Politics: Where Did it All Go Wrong?* Oxford: Firing the Mind.

Pinsky, E. (2011). The Olympian Delusion. *Journal of the American Psychoanalytic Association*, 59(2): 351–376.

Pinsky, E. (2014). The potion: Reflections on Freud's 'Observations on transference-love'. *Journal of the American Psychoanalytic Association*, 62: 455–474.

Pinsky, E. (2017). *Death and Fallibility in the Psychoanalytic Encounter: Mortal Gifts*. New York: Routledge.

Pirelli, G., Estoup, A., and Otto, R. K. (2016). Using Internet and social media data as collateral sources of information in forensic evaluations. *Professional Psychology, Research and Practice*, 47: 12–17.

Plato. *Meno*. G. M. A Grube (trans.). In: M. Cooper (ed.) (1997). *Plato, Complete Works*. Indiana: Hackett Publishing Company.

Poland, W. (2000). The analyst's witnessing and otherness. *Journal of the American Psychoanalytic Association*, 48(1): 17–34.

Pope, K., and Tabachnick, B. (1994). Therapists as patients: A national survey of psychologists' experiences, problems, and beliefs. *Professional Psychology: Research and Practice*, 25(3): 247–258.

Puget, J. (2017). Discussion of dominique Scarfone's Paper, 'On "That Is Not Psychoanalysis": Ethics as the main tool for psychoanalytic knowledge'. *Psychoanalytic Dialogues*, 27(4): 401–405.

Racker, H. (1957). The meanings and uses of countertransference. *Psychoanalytic Quarterly*, 26: 303–357.

Racker, H. (1968). *Transference and Countertransference*. New York: International University Press.

Radcliffe-Richards, J. (2012). *The Ethics of Transplants: Why Careless Thought Costs Lives*. Oxford: Oxford University Press.

Rapport, N. (2009). Ethics of apology. In: N. Mookherjee et al., (eds) *The Ethics of Apology: A Set of Commentaries. Critique of Anthropology*, 29(3): 345–366, London: Sage.

Rawls, J. (1973). *A Theory of Justice*. Oxford: Oxford University Press.

Reis, B. (2009). Performative and enactive features of psychoanalytic witnessing: The transference as the scene of address. *International Journal of Psychoanalysis*, 90: 1359–1372.

Renik, O. (1993). Analytic interaction: Conceptualising technique in light of the analyst's irreducible subjectivity. *Psychoanalytic Quarterly*, 62: 553–571.

Rilke, M. (1929). *Letters to a Young Poet*. London: Penguin.

Ringstrom, P. (1998). The pursuit of authenticity and the plight of self-deception: Commentary on paper by Slavin and Kriegman. *Psychoanalytic Dialogues*, 8(2): 285–292.

Roache, R. and Savulescu, J. (2018). Psychological disadvantage and a welfarist approach to psychiatry. *Philosophy, Psychiatry, & Psychology*, 25(4): 245–259.

Rokach, A. (2019). *The Psychological Journey to and from Loneliness: Development, Causes, and Effects of Social and Emotional Isolation*. Cambridge: Academic Press.

Ross, W. D. (1930). *The Right and the Good*. Oxford: Clarendon.

Rozmarin, E. (2007). An other in psychoanalysis: Emmanuel Levinas's critique of knowledge and analytic sense. *Contemporary Psychoanalysis*, 43: 327–360.

Rustin, M. (2001). *Reason and Unreason: Psychoanalysis, Science and Politics*. London: Continuum.

Saketopoulou, A. (2021). Does the sexual have anything to do with sexual boundary violations? In: Levin, C. (ed.) *Social Aspects of Sexual Boundary Trouble in Psychoanalysis, Responses to the Work of Muriel Dimen*. London: Routledge, pp. 101–128.

Savulescu, J. and Kahane, G. (2011). Disability: A welfarist approach. *Clinical Ethics*, 6(1): 45–51.

Savulescu, J., Sandberg, A., and Kahane, G. (2011). Well-being and enhancement. In: J. Savulescu, R. Meulen, and G. Kahane (eds) *Enhancing Human Capacities*. Oxford: Blackwell Publishing Ltd, pp. 1–18.

Savulescu, J. (1994). Rational desires and the limitation of life-sustaining treatment. *Bioethics*, 8: 191–222.

Scarfone, D. (2014). Preface. In: V. Chetrit-Vatine (ed.) *The Ethical Seduction of the Analytic Situation: The Feminine-Maternal Origins of Responsibility for the Other*. London: Karnac/Ipa.

Scarfone, D. (2017). On 'That Is Not Psychoanalysis': Ethics as the main tool for psychoanalytic knowledge and discussion. *Psychoanalytic Dialogues*, 27: 392–400.

Scarry, E. (1998). The Difficulty of Imagining Other People. In: E. Weiner (ed.) *The Handbook of Interethnic Coexistence*. New York: Continuum, pp. 40–62.

Schafer, R. (1994). A classic revisited:Kurt Eissler's 'The effect of the structure of the ego on psychoanalytic technique'. *International Journal of Psychoanalysis*, 75: 721–728.

Schonbar, R. (1986). The fee as a focus of transference and countertransference and treatment. In D. Kreuger (ed.) *The Last Taboo*. New York: Brunner/Mazel.

Shapiro, E. and Ginzberg, R. (2006). Buried treasure: Money, ethics, and counter-transference in group therapy. *International Journal of Group Psychotherapy*, 56(4): 477–494.

Shaull, R. (1996). *Introduction to Pedagogy of the Oppressed*. London: Penguin, 1996

Slavin, M. and Kriegman, D. (1998). Why the analyst needs to change: Toward a theory of conflict, negotiation, and mutual influence in the therapeutic process. *Psychoanalytic Dialogues*, 8(2): 247–284.

Slochower, J. (2003). The analyst's secret delinquencies. *Psychoanalytic Dialogues*, 13(4): 451–469.

Slochower, J. (2017). Don't tell anyone. *Psychoanalytic Psychology*, 34: 195–200.

Smith, C. and Freyd, J. (2014). Institutional betrayal. *American Psychologist*, 69: 575–587.

Smith, N. (2008). *I Was Wrong: The Meanings of Apologies*. Cambridge: Cambridge University Press.

Solomon, H. (2004). The ethical attitude in analytic training and practice. In: Joseph Cambray and Linda Carter (eds) *Analytical Psychology: Contemporary Perspectives in Jungian Analysis*. London: Brunner-Routledge, pp. 249–265.

Sousa, P., Pinheiro, R., and Silva, R. (2003). Questions about questions. *International Journal of Psychoanalysis*, 84: 865–878.

Sperber, D. and Wilson, D. (1986). *Relevance: Communication and Cognition* (1st ed.). Oxford: Blackwell.

Spillius, E. (2007). *Encounters with Melanie Klein: Selected Papers of Elizabeth Spillius*. London: Routledge.

Steiner, J. (1993). *Psychic Retreats: Pathological Organizations in Psychotic, Neurotic, and Borderline Patients*. London; New York: Routledge.

Steiner, J. (2000). Book review: A mind of one's own: A Kleinian view of self and object. By Robert Caper. London: Routledge. *Journal American Psychoanalytic Association*, 48(2): 637–643.

Stern, D. (2010). *Partners in Thought: Working with Unformulated Experience, Dissociation and Enactment*. London: Routledge.

Stolorow, R. D., Atwood, G. E., and Orange, D. M. (2002). *Worlds of Experience*. New York: Basic Books.

Suler, J. (2004). The online disinhibition effect. *Cyberpsychology & behavior*, 7(3): 321–326.

Symington, N. (1983). The analyst's act of freedom as agent of therapeutic change. *International Review of Psycho-Analysis*, 10(3): 283–291.

Taubman, P. (2010). Alain Badiou, Jacques Lacan and the ethics of teaching. *Educational Philosophy and Theory*, 42(2): 196–212.

Thornton, S. (2022). Practical irony: Reflections on a theme in the work of Jonathan Lear. *European Journal of Philosophy*, 30(2): 840–853.

Tuckett, D. (2000). Reporting clinical events in the journal: Towards the construction of a special case. *International Journal of Psychoanalysis*, 81: 1065–1069.

Tuckett, D. (2008). On differences, discussing differences and comparison. In: D. Tuckett, et al., (eds) *Psychoanalysis Comparable and Incomparable*. London: Routledge.

Tulipan, A. (1983). Fees in psychotherapy: A perspective. *Journal of the American Academy of Psychoanalysis*, 11: 445–463.

Tylim, I. (2005). The power of apologies in transforming resentment into forgiveness. *International Journal of Applied Psychoanalytic Studies*, 2(3): 260–270.

Van den Hoven, J. and Cocking, D. (2018). *Evil Online*. Chichester: Wiley-Blackwell.

Vincent, N. (2013). *Neuroscience and Legal Responsibility*. Nicole A. Vincent (ed.) New York: Oxford University Press.

Vines, P. (2007). The power of apology: Mercy, forgiveness or corrective justice in the civil liability arena. *Public Space: The Journal of Law and Social Justice*, 1(1): 14.

Vodanovich, S., Sundaram, D., and Myers, M. (2010). Research commentary: Digital natives and ubiquitous information. *Information Systems Research*, 21: 711–723.

Walaszewska, E. and Piskorska, A. (2012). *Relevance Theory: More than Understanding*. Cambridge: Cambridge Scholars.

Wallwork, E. (1991). *Psychoanalysis and Ethics*. New Haven: Yale University Press.

Ware, O. (2009). The duty of self-knowledge. *Philosophy and Phenomenological Research*, 79(3): 671–698.

Watson, L. (2018). Systematic epistemic rights violations in the media: A Brexit case study. *Social Epistemology*, 32(2): 88–102.

Weil, S. (1952). *The Need for Roots: Prelude to a Declaration of Duties Towards Mankind*. Routledge and Kegan Paul.

Welfel, E. (2015). Ethics in counselling & psychotherapy. Boston, MA: Cengage Learning.

Wild, J. (1969). Introduction. In: Levinas, E. (ed.) *Totality and Infinity: An Essay on Exteriority*. Pittsburgh: Duquesne University Press, pp. 1–10.

Williams, B. (1981). Moral Luck. In: *Moral Luck: Philosophical Papers 1973–80*. Cambridge: Cambridge University Press, pp. 20–39.

Wilson, M. (2012). The flourishing analyst, responsibility, and psychoanalytic ethics. *Journal of the American Psychoanalytic Association*, 60(6): 1251–1258.

Wilson, M. (2013). Desire and responsibility: The ethics of countertransference experience. *The Psychoanalytic Quarterly*, 82(2): 435–476.

Wilson, M. (2020). *The Analyst's Desire: The Ethical Foundation of Clinical Practice (Psychoanalytic Horizons)*. London: Bloomsbury.

Winnicott, D. W. (1949). Hate in the countertransference. *International Journal of Psychoanalysis*, 30: 69–67.

Winnicott, D. W. (1969). The use of an object. *International Journal of Psychoanalysis*, 50: 711–716.

Wood, H. (2011). The Internet and its role in the escalation of sexually compulsive behaviour. *Psychoanalytic Psychotherapy*, 25(2): 127–142.

Wren, B. (2019). Ethical issues arising in the provision of medical interventions for gender diverse children and adolescents. *Clinical Child Psychology and Psychiatry*, 24(2): 203–222.

Zohny, H., Earp, B., and Savulescu, J. (2022). Enhancing gender. *Journal of Bioethical Inquiry*, 19(2), 225–237.

Subject Index